MEDIEVAL DISABILITY HERITAGE

COLLECTION DEVELOPMENT, CULTURAL HERITAGE, AND DIGITAL HUMANITIES

Further Information and Publications

www.arc-humanities.org/series/book-series/

MEDIEVAL DISABILITY HERITAGE

THE MUSEUM EXHIBITION REIMAGINED

by

KISHA G. TRACY

ARC HUMANITIES PRESS

British Library Cataloguing in Publication Data
A catalogue record for this book is available from the British Library.

ISBN (Hardback): 9781802703597
e-ISBN (PDF): 9781802705157
e-ISBN (ePUB): 9781802705164

DOI: 10.17302/asgs3268

www.arc-humanities.org

Printed and bound in the UK (by CPIGroup [UK] Ltd), USA (by Bookmasters), and elsewhere using print-on-demand technology.

Publisher (manufacturer) details: Arc Humanities Press, 14 Clifton Moor Business Village, James Nicolson Link, York YO30 4XG, United Kingdom.

EU Authorized Representative details (for GPSR purposes): Amsterdam University Press, Nieuwe Prinsengracht 89, 1018 VR Amsterdam, The Netherlands. www.aup.nl

To my mother,
whose curiosity and kindness
inspires me daily

To my husband, Chris,
whose support and love
means everything to me

To my younger self,
for whom it would have been difficult to imagine
that this life would be possible

CONTENTS

DOI: 10.17302/asgs32681 © Arc Humanities Press

LIST OF ILLUSTRATIONS

DOI: 10.17302/asgs32682 © Arc Humanities Press

PREFACE

I WOULD LIKE to acknowledge that I am a white, tenured professor who identifies as a woman and a person with a disability. I recognize the vital significance of studying the global Middle Ages and marginalized communities. I am sensitive to the fact that, as a white woman whose primary training is in Middle English, I perhaps am not always the ideal person to teach this material, in terms of experience, in terms of demonstrating representation, and in terms of my space of privilege. However, I am committed to actively doing my best to seek ways to amplify different perspectives, in research and in classrooms, and the scholars who know far more than I on these subjects.

There has been a great deal of ongoing discussion about the appropriateness of the term "medieval" for non-European regions in this premodern period. The field and adjacent ones, however, have as yet not come to a consensus about a replacement term, so I will continue to use "medieval" in this book.[1]

Unless otherwise noted, references to the sex of individuals are biological only. We cannot always know the lived experience of gender of these individuals.

1 See Holmes and Standen, "Introduction," for a discussion of this topic.

DOI: 10.17302/asgs32683 © Arc Humanities Press

INTRODUCTION

THIS INTERDISCIPLINARY EXPLORATION of medieval disability is arranged into sections on how bodies tell stories, the daily lives of people with disabilities, and making the intangible tangible. It seeks to shed new light on the use and interrogation of available source materials of all kinds, to articulate pressing themes in disability studies, and to foreground the importance of visibility and inclusivity. The book is influenced by guides to museum exhibitions, suggesting an imagined exhibition about medieval disability cultural heritage that is not bound by the logistics or the physical space of an actual museum. I will discuss this approach more at the end of the introduction, but, first, we will begin by introducing the concepts of cultural heritage and medieval and disability heritage.

Medieval Cultural Heritage

In the late ninth century, King Alfred the Great, in his Old English preface to a translation of Pope Gregory's *Pastoral Care*, laments the loss of cultural heritage in his country. He states, in translation, "I also remembered how I saw, before it had all been ravaged and burnt, how the churches throughout all England stood filled with treasures and books."[1] While Alfred is looking back to a mostly legendary past, his concern for the loss of previous heritage demonstrates a sense of its value and the disadvantages indicated by its destruction. Alfred is by far not the only premodern person to lament the loss of cultural heritage and to advocate for its preservation. The need to preserve and explanations of why to do so are common in the premodern eras, and this tradition has continued into the modern era, in which we now see international laws and organizations dedicated to preservation.

1 "Translation of Alfred's Prose Preface to Pastoral Care."

DOI: 10.17302/asgs32684 © Arc Humanities Press

What Is Cultural Heritage?

First, we need to establish a definition of cultural heritage. In its glossary, the United Nations Educational, Scientific, and Cultural Organization (UNESCO) provides the following:

> Cultural heritage includes artefacts, monuments, a group of buildings and sites, museums that have a diversity of values including symbolic, historic, artistic, aesthetic, ethnological or anthropological, scientific and social significance. It includes tangible heritage (movable, immobile and underwater), intangible cultural heritage (ICH) embedded into cultural, and natural heritage artefacts, sites or monuments.[2]

The "diversity of values" listed in this definition illustrates the range of meanings that heritage can have. The Harvard University Department of History of Art and Architecture's "Whose Culture? The Curation and Management of World Heritage" project further refines this definition:

> [heritage] is a generational inheritance, one which may be either tangible or intangible. Intangible forms of heritage include oral traditions, community bonds, and language. Tangible forms of heritage are...material traces left behind which transmit important cultural and historical knowledge from one generation to the next.

There is an emphasis here on "inheritance" that is passed down through generations in order to preserve "cultural and historical knowledge." This leads us to ask: What happens when important heritage is destroyed or deliberately erased?

Medieval Material Culture and Intangible Heritage

Objects are more than physical, inanimate "things." Julie Lund and Sarah Semple argue that material culture is a "rich stepping-off point for understanding time and memory, the lived experience, sensory worlds and engagements, embodiment, and the medieval life course."[3] Cultural objects have stories and histories of their own, particularly as imbued in them by the humans who created and interacted with them, giving them meaning and significance. In addition, the "fact that objects and structures may endure longer than human beings may provide them with the potential to act as time marks: things that can hold and carry memories, stories, and myths."[4]

---

2 UNESCO, "Cultural Heritage."

3 Lund and Semple, "Introduction," 1.

4 Lund and Semple, "Introduction," 5.

Medieval people were well aware of the role of objects in carrying and transmitting meaning as well as even a sense of identity and place.

Some of the most revered objects in the European Middle Ages were relics. These were the "physical remains of a holy site or holy person, or objects with which they had contact," and the "containers that store and display relics" are reliquaries, themselves usually made from valuable materials.[5] The idea of relics stems from the perception of holy bodies, such as those of saints, as sacred and incorruptible. Initially, only parts of the body like hair and nails were removed, as these were considered to be unnecessary in the afterlife.[6] In other instances, when body parts were separated from a holy person in life—for example, decapitations—they also could be preserved and turned into relics.[7] These rules, however, began to shift in the ninth and tenth centuries: "Whereas originally the saint and his sacred power could be manifested only in a complete body, they could now be manifested in individual parts as well. Veneration was accorded to them as to the whole body, and so we can speak of a 'real presence of the saints in their relics.'"[8] Garments and other objects that came into contact with holy individuals also had the same, if slightly lower, special place. There was a concern about the validity of relics, and there were methods to try to authenticate them, including "especially certificates of authenticity, finger-wide strips of parchment with the saint's name, or even the fire test, since relics were considered not to be flammable."[9] While authenticity was certainly a concern in the Middle Ages, in terms of heritage the reverence given to these objects is more essential than whether they are indeed real. Later in the Middle Ages, relics became public objects, placed on view for veneration and visitation.[10]

There is perhaps no clearer metaphor for the significance placed on cultural heritage in the Middle Ages than the chained library. Popular until the eighteenth century, these libraries used chains to attach the cover of each book to the shelf, allowing a reader to move the book from the shelf to the desk in front of it, but not to remove it from the library. Such a system ensured the security of the books and a desire to protect the collections,

---

5 Boehm, "Relics and Reliquaries."

6 Angenendt, "Relics and Their Veneration," 22.

7 Angenendt, "Relics and Their Veneration," 23.

8 Angenendt, "Relics and Their Veneration," 23.

9 Angenendt, "Relics and Their Veneration," 23.

10 See Chapter 1's "Contexts: Ethics of Displaying the Human Body" on the idea of human remains as heritage.

especially from theft. The Hereford Cathedral Chained Library is the largest still in existence, with all its chains and locks, and its oldest book is the eighth-century *Hereford Gospels*.[11]

While the books themselves are tangible heritage, what they represent and the knowledge within them are intangible. As Lars Boje Mortensen writes, "texts can be said to live a life at a somewhat indeterminate point between the material and the abstract realms."[12] Further, Mortensen makes a case for officially naming what books contain and disseminate as intangible cultural heritage, due to "(1) the specific textual fluidity before printing, (2) our distance to the relevant main languages, (3) the disproportionate weight of the textual record in understanding the distant past."[13] The transmission history of many medieval manuscripts, the ramifications of translation, and the important role of written text both emphasize abstractness as well as how essential manuscripts are to medieval heritage.

Cultural Heritage at Risk

As noted by Alfred the Great, cultural heritage is fragile. There are multiple factors that can contribute to its damage or destruction, some intentional and others accidental. For example, it is startling to consider just how many manuscripts have been lost. Using the statistical "unseen species model," of the medieval European manuscripts written in English, French, Dutch, German, Irish, and Icelandic on narrative and chivalric fiction that likely existed, it is possible that about 89.9% have disappeared.[14]

Cultural heritage is particularly vulnerable in times of war. Alberto Frigerio, in his article "Heritage Under Attack: A Critical Analysis of the Reasons Behind the Destruction of Cultural Property in the Event of Armed Conflict," cites "the most common reasons that have led to the intentional destruction of cultural property in the last 25 years [as] military necessity, psychological warfare, inter-ethnic hatred, religious radicalism, and planned/opportunistic looting," stating that "the clashing forces have intentionally attacked the cultural property to whom their rivals were emotionally tied in order to gain certain psychological effect."[15] The two World Wars were, in particular, devastating for medieval heritage. The library of KU Leuven—a Catholic

11 Hereford Cathedral, "Chained Library."

12 Mortensen, "Why Ancient and Medieval Texts Are Intangible Cultural Heritage."

13 See Chapter 3 for more on oral storytelling.

14 Kestemont et al., "Forgotten Books," 768.

15 Frigerio, "Heritage Under Attack."

university in Leuven, Belgium, originally called Universitas Lovaniensis and founded in 1425—was sacked and burned by the Germans in 1914 at the beginning of WWI; upon its destruction, "close to one thousand manuscripts and about 800 incunables...lost in a blaze that lasted ten hours."[16] This is only one incident in the library's history. As their website lists, they were "bombed by the French in 1797, burned down by German troops in 1914 and again in 1940, and finally split up in 1970"; yet, they are proud of the fact that "each time the university library rose like the proverbial phoenix from its ashes."[17]

The loss of cultural heritage at Leuven was a tragic casualty of war, but there are also instances in which heritage is specifically targeted. Discussing the ongoing war in Ukraine, Glòria Munilla comments that "[h]eritage is a basic tool for attacking the foundations of a cultural group's culture and identity. Its systematic, conscious and deliberate destruction is part of the strategies of war."[18] As a further example, in 2022 the Caucasus Heritage Watch (CHW) reported that in the Nakhchivan Autonomous Republic of Azerbaijan during the Second Nagorno-Karabakh War there was "the complete destruction of 108 medieval and early modern Armenian monasteries, churches, and cemeteries between 1997 and 2011," which "represents 98% of the Armenian cultural heritage sites" they investigated.[19] The Nagorno-Karabakh region is contested by Azerbaijan, Armenia, and Artsakh, and ethnic violence has erupted on multiple occasions. The CHW report dubs the destruction of this medieval Armenian heritage as "silent and systematic cultural erasure" that "has been a feature of Azerbaijan's domestic ethnic policies." Targeting heritage is a way to attack the identity of a culture.

Medieval heritage in Europe has in particular been the victim of iconoclasm—the destruction of sacred or venerable objects or representations—especially during the Protestant Reformation and the English Dissolution of the Monasteries. The word *iconoclasm* derives from the Greek *eikon* (image) and *klan* (to break), thus literally meaning "image-breaking." Acts of iconoclasm are very old. According to the Maxwell Museum of Anthropology's guide to the exhibition "Iconoclasm: Questions of Veneration, Destruction and Power," "As long as humans have created symbols, others have sought to

16 Hoeniger, "The English Gift After the Destruction of the University of Louvain Library," 85.

17 KU Leuven, "History of the University Library."

18 Iglesias, "Destruction of Cultural Heritage."

19 Caucasus Heritage Watch, "Silent Erasure."

destroy them, creating cycles of veneration and destruction."[20] In the eighth to the ninth centuries in Byzantium, there was a theological debate about iconoclasm that led to the removal or destruction of religious imagery in response to the Bible's exhortation not to worship idols:

> How could a piece of wood painted with a figure channel a believer's prayers to the saint portrayed? What was the difference between honouring an icon and worshipping a pagan idol, which the second commandment—which reads: "Thou shalt not make to thyself an idol, nor likeness of anything... Thou shalt not bow down to them, nor serve them..." (Exodus 20:4–5)—clearly prohibited?[21]

This belief is echoed in the Protestant Reformation of the sixteenth century. Distressed by the excesses of the Catholic Church and fuelled by anxieties about idols, Protestants destroyed many statues, paintings, and other objects in churches around Europe. Relics also received their ire, and "the Calvinists congratulated themselves that no saints had resisted when they destroyed the images of the saints or when they burned their relics."[22] Iconoclasm is generally done in the belief that the destruction is necessary:

> The iconoclasts, on the other hand, whether we are talking about ancient Christians, sixteenth century Protestants zealots (who destroyed statues and stained glass windows that were masterpieces), the Taliban, or indeed the Serbians in Bosnia and Kosovo, always justify their actions, and always convince themselves that what they are doing is not only necessary but just.[23]

We have seen further examples of iconoclasm in the Black Lives Matter movement and in the destruction of Confederate and Columbus statues. All these instances are intended as commentary on systemic social issues.

Since so much cultural heritage is flammable, fire is one of its natural enemies. Prior to (and even after) the invention of gunpowder and machines of war, fire was a primary method of razing cities, but it is also an accidental means of destruction. One of the most famous accidental fires in the destruction of medieval heritage was in 1731 at Ashburnham House in Westminster, England, damaging the collection known as the Cotton Library. The library was collected by antiquarian Sir Robert Bruce Cotton, who lived 1571–1631, and it had been gifted to the British crown in 1701 by his descendant, Sir John Cotton. The damage was extensive: "It fatally damaged a copy of the *Magna*

---

20 Maxwell Museum of Anthropology, "Iconoclasm."

21 Brubaker, *Inventing Byzantine Iconoclasm*, 22.

22 Angenendt, "Relics and Their Veneration," 26.

23 Dwyer, "Destroying the Past."

Carta and scarred the only known text of *Beowulf*, entirely destroying Asser's ninth-century biography of King Alfred and a fifth-century Greek Genesis, among other works."[24] Looking at the scarring on the *Beowulf* manuscript is an emotional experience, starkly emphasizing the ephemeral nature of many types of heritage.

The Preservation of Cultural Heritage

Tomas Nilson and Kristina Thorell identify four main reasons for the preservation of cultural heritage: "(1) scientific (research and increased knowledge), (2) political (messages and symbolism), (3) social (sense of place and cultural identity) and (4) economic (attracts tourists and visitors to the region)."[25] Twelfth-century English chronicler and Benedictine monk Orderic Vitalis, in his *Ecclesiastical History*, emphasizes the first, knowledge, and the third, identity:

> without books the deeds of the ancients pass into oblivion and can in no way be recovered by us moderns, for the admonitions of the men of old pass away from the memory of the present with the changing world, as hail or snow melt in the waters of a swift river, swept away by the current, never to return.[26]

Alfred, in his preface to the *Pastoral Care*, comments on losing the benefits of knowledge due to an inability to understand the languages of previous texts: "And they had very little benefit from those books, for they could not understand anything in them, because they were not written in their own language...we have now lost both the wealth and the wisdom, because we would not bend down to their tracks with our minds." Medieval texts on art technologies also indicate a concern with damage and repair, offering recipes for ways to prolong durability or fix artworks.[27]

Orderic, Alfred, and these other authors would likely be advocates for what we now call heritage preservation.

In the intervening centuries, many have contributed to the preservation of medieval heritage. The lengths to which the librarians went to try to save as much of the Cotton Library as they were able are laudable. The American Bookbinders Museum notes a copy of the report to Parliament after the incident:

---

24 Burgess, "Time's Teeth," 303.

25 Nilson and Thorell, *Cultural Heritage Preservation*, 12.

26 Orderic Vitalis, *Historia Ecclesiastics*, ed. Chibnall, vol. 3, p. 284; Clanchy, "Tenacious Letters," 116.

27 Van Daal, "Prevention, Breakage, Care."

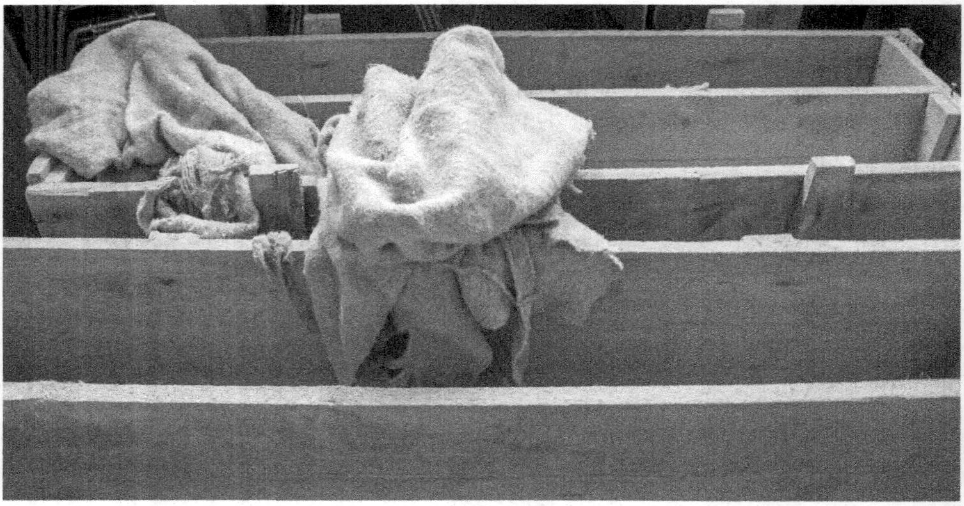

Figure 1. Replica crates holding artworks. Nuremberg Historischer Kunstbunker. Nuremberg, Germany. Photograph by author.

> Mr. Casley, the Deputy Librarian, took Care in the First Place to remove the famous Alexandrian MS. and the Books under the Head of Augustus in the Cottonian Library, as being esteemed the most valuable amongst the Collection. Several intire [*sic*] Presses** with the Books in them were also removed; but the Fire increasing still, and the Engines sent for not coming so soon as could be wished, and several of the Backs of the Presses being already on Fire, they were obliged to be broke [*sic*] open, and the Books, as many as could be, were thrown out of the Windows.[28]

We have much to thank Mr. Casley for in terms of preserving what he could.

We also have the Monuments, Fine Arts, and Archives Section Unit (MFAA), also known as the Monuments Men and Women, to thank for the preservation of medieval heritage at risk in World War II. It is well documented how the Nazis collected and looted cultural treasures in all of the countries that they invaded. Heinrich Himmler, the head of the SS and creator of the research organization Ahnenerbe, or "ancestral heritage," was particularly obsessed with the past.[29] The artifacts they took were sent back to Germany, often finding their way into bunkers, like that in the city of

28 American Bookbinders Museum, "The Cottonian Library Fire."

29 For more on Himmler's obsession with the Middle Ages, see Diebold, "The Nazi Middle Ages."

Nuremberg, to protect them and German treasures from Allied air raids.[30] The Monuments Men and Women located these hiding places and recovered priceless works. In Nuremberg's Historischer Kunstbunker (see Fig. 1), which can be explored today, they found the fifteenth-century altar by Veit Stoss from Saint Mary's Church in Kraków, Poland, as well as the Imperial Insignia of the Holy Roman Empire. The Smithsonian Archives of American Art has a number of oral interviews with members of the MFAA detailing their exploits in their own words.[31]

The Pros and Cons of Reproductions and Digitization

The discussion of the pros and cons of copies goes back at least as far as Platonic realism. John Berger's *Ways of Seeing* recognizes that reproductions democratize art by allowing everyone access to it, but, at the same time, he argues that they lack the gravitas and the presence of the originals. Clive Bell writes:

> A literal copy is seldom reckoned even by its owner a work of art. It leaves us cold; its forms are not significant. Yet if it were an absolutely exact copy, clearly it would be as moving as the original, and a photographic reproduction of a drawing often is—almost. Evidently, it is impossible to imitate a work of art exactly; and the differences between the copy and the original, minute though they may be, exist and are felt immediately.[32]

To expand this concept to all forms of cultural heritage, perhaps it is that the original has experiences that are impossible to replicate, rather like individual humans themselves. The circumstances of its creation, its day-to-day existence, the people who have interacted with it, its struggle for preservation make it unique.

On the other hand, increased access is important. Not everyone can travel to see cultural objects in person or study manuscripts in a major library collection. In terms of manuscripts, Martin Foys says that they are not fixed objects:

> The surviving physical manuscript only inconsistently records and retains the changes it has undergone over centuries, while the scholarship and scholarly resources that surround the manuscript have tended to do the

30 See Chapter 3 for a discussion of the Canterbury Cathedral stained glass that survived WWII in England.

31 Smithsonian Archives of American Art, "Monuments Men Series."

32 Bell, "Art," 52–53.

> same, selectively reproducing its matter through other media formats, first in print, and now increasingly in digital.[33]

Given that a manuscript—or any cultural object—has many lives, a reproduction or a digital copy is only another one of those lives. It is in the interaction with readers or viewers or researchers that its significance is continued.

An example of this value of reproduction is Notre Dame Cathedral in Paris, France, which experienced a major fire on April 15, 2019. After the smoke had cleared, discussions of how or if to rebuild it started. Four years prior to this disaster, Professor of Art Andrew Tallon had created a "spatial map of Notre Dame using more than a billion laser-measured points," which allowed for a digital replica of the cathedral.[34] While Tallon himself did not get to see it, as he passed away, his work was used in helping to rebuild Notre Dame. Philippe Villeneuve, Architect-in-Chief of Historic Monuments in charge of the cathedral's preservation, stated that Tallon's "scan enabled us to reconstruct the vaults without any hesitation from a dimensional or formal standpoint, and it also granted us total freedom to understand how [the cathedral] was made, to be able to rebuild it in a thoughtful, intellectual, and intelligent way."[35] The digital replica made possible by Andrew Tallon may not have unto itself the heritage of the original cathedral, but its existence gave another life to the cultural treasure, illustrating the value of reproduction.

Medieval Disability Cultural Heritage

Nathaniel Vincent Mohatt et al. define "historical trauma" as that which "refers to a complex and collective trauma experienced over time and across generations by a group of people who share an identity, affiliation, or circumstance."[36] The Substance Abuse and Mental Health Services Administration previously identified it as "often associated with racial and ethnic population groups...who have suffered major intergenerational losses and assaults on their culture and well-being."[37] People with disabilities are such a community, with their heritage forgotten (either consciously or unconsciously) or sensationalized. The study and sharing of disability

33 Foys, "Medieval Manuscripts," 119.

34 Lou, "Four Years Ago, An Art Historian Used Lasers."

35 Cook, "Leaving a Trace."

36 Mohatt et al., "Historical Trauma as Public Narrative," 129.

37 "Trauma and Violence."

heritage allows for a restoration of historical well-being. As we noted before, Nilson and Thorell identify the social, a sense of place and cultural identity, as a reason for preserving cultural heritage. This, along with scientific research, gives clear impetuses for disability heritage both to increase knowledge and to support a sense of identity in a marginalized community.[38]

Medieval Disability

Modern conceptions about historical disability tend to be exclusively pessimistic, reinforced by images in various types of media. This oversimplified representation is supported by misconceptions of the Middle Ages as a whole and the perpetuation of the "Dark Ages" myth. The popular perception of this time period is tainted by grey film filters and grim storylines, usually involving the plague. This monolithic, negative image of the Middle Ages spills over into representations of disability; people with disabilities are relegated to victims of mistreatment and symbols of the supposed excessive violence of this era.

In reality, the Middle Ages were a vibrant and complex time, filled with diverse human beings living their lives, experiencing both the highs and lows of existence.[39] The same is true for medieval people with disabilities. While there are examples of negative treatment, there are also examples of positive experiences and, perhaps even more telling, neutral experiences that indicate there were circumstances in which disability was treated as an ordinary part of life.

Medieval Disability Cultural Heritage

Cultural heritage can help us understand the role of disability in the Middle Ages. The connection between material culture and disability moves it from an abstract concept to a concrete reality:

> The relationship between material culture and disability can be viewed as a fundamental one, as material culture does not only provide aids, but it can furthermore contribute to cultural conceptions around disability (Ott 2018). Take for example, the current symbolic role of the wheelchair as a universal emblem for disability access (International Symbol of Access) or the effects of a wider access to eyeglasses to a changed perception of visual impairment.[40]

---

38 Nilson and Thorell, *Cultural Heritage Preservation*, 12.

39 See Tracy, *Why Study the Middle Ages?*.

40 Sveinsdóttir, "A Material Culture of Medieval Disability," 47.

Material culture emphasizes the significance of the visibility of disability cultural heritage and the necessity to interpret heritage through the lens of disability.

For instance, the cultural heritage of medieval disability includes the Bible, undeniably heritage in its own right. The Bible has contributed to the perceptions of disability for centuries and is an important text for the European Middle Ages. There are multiple references to disability in the Bible, some associating it with charity, others with sin, but one in Exodus is particularly significant: "The Lord said to him: Who made man's mouth? or who made the dumb and the deaf, the seeing and the blind? did not I? (Exodus 4:11)."[41] In this passage, God tells Moses that people with disabilities were created by divine order and are thus in a sense special and protected. Reading the Bible through a disability lens, and particularly from the perspective of the people of the Middle Ages, gives us access to these cultural conceptions.

STORIES: Examining a Coin of John the Blind

To illustrate how this might work, we can look at the example of a coin minted during the time of John the Blind's reign in Bohemia, which lasted from 1310–1346. Son of Holy Roman Emperor Henry VII, John was born in Luxembourg and was married to Elizabeth of Bohemia, daughter of Wenceslaus II. After their marriage, John invaded Bohemia, deposing the king, Henry of Gorizia, making himself unpopular in Czechoslovakia.[42] In 1336, John went blind as a result of ophthalmia—an inflammation of the eye. He was, however, still active for ten years before his death in 1346 at the Battle of Crécy in the Hundred Years' War. The chronicler Jean Froissart describes John's final moments in the battle:

> for all that he was nigh blind, when he understood the order of the battle, he said to the [men] about him: "Where is the lord Charles my son?" His men said: "Sir we cannot tell; we think he be fighting." Then he said: "Sirs, ye are my men, my companions and friends in this journey: I require you bring me so far forward, that I may strike one stroke with my sword." They said they would do his commandment, and to the intent that they should not lose him in the press, they tied all their reins of their bridles each to other and set

---

41 All translations of the Bible are from the Douay-Rheims. Note the use of archaic language now considered offensive. See *Douay-Rheims Bible Online*, https://www.drbo.org.

42 For biographical information, see Agnew, *The Czechs and the Lands of the Bohemian Crown*.

> the king before to accomplish his desire, and so they went on their enemies. The lord Charles of Bohemia his son, who wrote himself king of Almaine and bare the arms, he came in good order to the battle; but when he saw that the matter went awry on their party, he departed, I cannot tell you which way. The king his father was so far forward that he strake a stroke with his sword, yea and more than four, and fought valiantly and so did his company; and they adventured themselves so forward, that they were there all slain; and the next day they were found in the place about the king, and all their horses tied each to other.[43]

This passage by Froissart highlights first John's disability, then his own response to it, which is to continue his activities as a king and as a military leader. It also emphasizes the loyalty of his men, their willingness to support him and accommodate his disability to the point of sacrificing their own lives. Indeed, John has become, as one business site indicates, "intrinsic to Luxembourg's collective identity."[44]

The physical artifacts that remain of many rulers are the coins minted during their reigns. Coins are recognized as a form of cultural heritage, serving "as the very essence of identity, unveiling all historical and geographical facets, transcending to shed light on artistic characteristics, religious beliefs, economic values, and political significance."[45] Thus, a Bohemian silver *Groschen* (coin) from the reign of John (see Fig. 2) is unto itself cultural heritage, but it is also indicative of the life of John the Blind and his role as a disabled monarch as he continued to rule and administer his kingdom. As such, it is part of medieval disability cultural heritage as well.

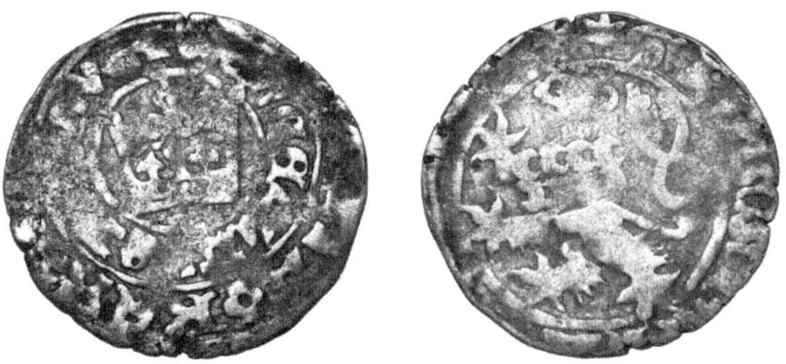

Figure 2. Bohemian silver *Groschen* of John the Blind, 1310–1346. Photograph by author.

43 Froissart, "Jean Froissart."

44 Decision Makers of Luxembourg, "John the Blind."

45 Kharoubi and Badra, "Importance of Coins in Historical and Archaeological Studies," 255.

"Stories" like this one are interspersed throughout this book, at the end of each section. These are intended to provide focused insights into particular examples of medieval disability heritage, and to illustrate artifacts with multiple levels of heritage significance such as the Coin of John the Blind or, on p. 30, the discovery of Richard III; the heritage about which we have more ambiguous evidence, such as Egil Skallagrímsson's legendary skull (see p. 43); and those with modern connections, such as the Saint Clare Garden (see p. 93).

Incomplete Representations

Although we have much in the way of evidence about medieval disability, its representation in cultural spaces is still limited and often does not address any of its complexities or depth. An exhibit at the Morgan Library and Museum, "Medieval Monsters: Terrors, Aliens, Wonders," categorized people with disabilities under "Aliens," emphasizing the connection between the disabled and the monstrous. While this connection certainly existed, it is far from the only medieval representation. The Getty Museum exhibition "Outcasts: Prejudice and Persecution in the Medieval World" included a section on "Ableism and Classism," focusing on the role of the disabled in charity and how they were often satirized. Again, these are valid experiences to emphasize, but focusing on them to the exclusion of all other representations does not do justice to a full understanding of disability in the Middle Ages.

The Problem of Sources

An issue that must be contended with in the study of historic disability is the different types of sources that need to be consulted or collected in addition to the traditional written records that medieval disability studies scholars tend to analyze, ones that have been privileged for generations. In Africa, we have archaeological evidence of pottery and figures depicting certain medieval legendary and historical individuals who represent disability; thus we have visual sources to consider. For instance, the Metropolitan Museum holds an *oba* (or mask) depicting Idia, an *iyoba* (or queen-mother) of Benin at the end of the fifteenth century, with "[t]wo vertical bars of inlaid iron between the eyes allude to medicine-filled incisions that were one source of Idia's metaphysical power."[46] This mask is an example of the heritage of healing. In addition, when written texts do exist, they have not received a great deal of attention. Consoler Teboh observes with respect to mental health in Africa, "Although

46 Bortolot, "Women Leaders in African History."

precolonial writings and oral histories covering centuries of the continent's history have survived (Understanding Slavery, 2011), it is unknown how many of these works address mental illness."[47] This assessment suggests that these sources have not been sufficiently analyzed in terms of disability.

Curation and Heritage Spaces

Curation is a powerful tool and a useful skill. It allows us to emphasize specific topics or ideas. It is particularly helpful in heritage spaces to narrow down the vast range of human stories. There are different types of heritage spaces. Museums are perhaps the most well-known as collectors, curators, and preservers of culture as well as spaces that educate the general public. They are not without their problems, however. Museums tend to be beholden to those who finance them, whether that is the state or a private entity. Many also have controversial histories, as in the problematic collection practices of the British Museum. In recent years, there have been many discussions about the repatriation of artifacts stolen from colonized lands and peoples. In addition, to see the cultural heritage in museums in person may require travel, depending on where a person lives, which requires the funding and ability to do so. Other physical spaces can be found in various venues: historical societies, universities, and libraries, among others.

The virtual world has become a popular space for heritage, which does address the accessibility issue if not the question of the original versus copies or digitization. These spaces allow for an easier dissemination of heritage to larger audiences, and they can avoid some of the issues related to patronage or ownership. They, however, rely on reproductions in the form of photographs and illustrations, and at times they suffer from a loosening of standards in terms of contextualization.

One of the benefits of curation is the ability to make visible heritage that is often marginalized or erased. Maura Reilly, in *Curatorial Activism: Towards an Ethics of Curating*, discusses how curation can both reinforce traditional marginalization by continuing to exclude certain people or it can resist this erasure by choosing to showcase and keep space for these voices.[48] That this resistance is, as Reilly defines it, an act of activism has become even more apparent in the United States in 2025, when heritage spaces are under pressure to remove content about diversity, including women, queer people, non-whites, and, indeed, those with disabilities.

---

47 Teboh, "Mental Health Inequities in Africa," 193.

48 See Reilly, *Curatorial Activism.*

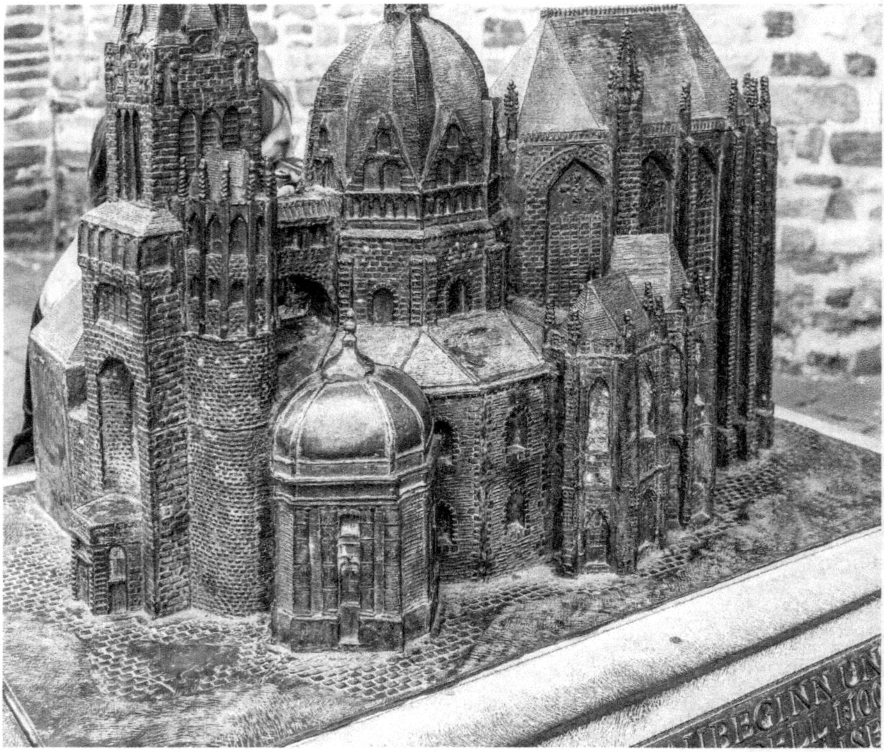

Figure 3. Egbert Broerken model of Aachen Cathedral.
Aachen, Germany. Photograph by author.

Accessibility to the Medieval

As purveyors of our collective story, all cultural heritage spaces should consider accessibility. Disability cultural heritage provides a unique opportunity to ally accessibility with content, but it should be a consideration no matter the subject.

Examples of accessibility at medieval sites are the tactile models of cultural buildings for the visually impaired by Egbert Broerken. According to his website, Broerken began creating these models over twenty years ago. They present whole towns or buildings, including Braille descriptions and explanations. Figure 3 shows the one at Aachen Cathedral in Germany. As his site states, these models are tactile ways for those with visual impairments to experience this heritage: "For this first time they can make an [architectural], historical or touristy experience in three dimensions."[49] Given the

49 Broerken, "Take a Walk Through the Streets on Your Fingertips."

scale of some of these buildings and towns, even the sighted are likely to discover details in the models that they otherwise might have missed.[50]

About this Volume

This book presents a selection of artifacts that I have "curated" to form an imaginary museum exhibition. In the process of choosing these pieces of heritage, I focused on breadth of significance. Each item not only tells us about its own story but also opens up discussions about larger aspects of disability and the study of disability.

It builds on the benefits of both physical and virtual spaces by conceptualizing the pieces as an imagined exhibition. Making the most of this conceptual space, which is unbound by the limitations of physical space, it does not confine itself to any particular type of artifact but encompasses collections of every kind: oral storytelling, locations, even whole cities. Its format is influenced by museum interpretations and exhibition guides, providing the context necessary for individuals to make connections beyond the limits of each specific artifact.

There are many other ways this space could be organized, and many other pieces of cultural heritage that could be included. Readers should consider how they could expand or revise this collection. In addition, it is productive to think about how we might translate this or other imaginary exhibitions into other types of spaces, whether digitally effected or situated beyond the museum's walls in other ways, to prioritize accessibility and underrepresented heritages.

---

50 See Stewart, "Mini Sculptures in Front of Monuments."

Chapter 1

THE BODY TELLS A STORY

AS WE BEGIN our exploration of this imagined exhibition, we might envision a series of dig sites with archaeological gear—trowels, shovels, sieves, notebooks, survey equipment, etc.—strewn about.

Section 1: Archaeological Discoveries

Archaeological discoveries have been instrumental in illuminating the lives of medieval people with disabilities. Bioarchaeology helps to reveal the stories that human remains have to tell, giving us insight into their daily lives. Osteobiography puts the pieces of these stories together and has already proved its value in providing "'a past with faces,' a past in which all people, rather than just textually privileged ones, have humanity and agency rather than remaining 'faceless blobs.'"[1] These fields reveal uniqueness and diversity, looking at human remains as individuals and introducing us to their lived experiences.

Knife-Hand Prosthesis

Longobard, Italy, sixth to eighth centuries

Upon discovery of a skeleton in Longobard, Italy, archaeologists realized that the forty to fifty-year-old male had an unexpected feature: a knife-hand prosthetic (see Fig. 4). The hand was bent over the man's stomach. Due to the way it was positioned and because of the wear on the arm and what remains of it, the archaeologists deduced that the knife was a prosthetic that he used in daily life. Further, upon study of the man's teeth, they found dental wear that indicated regular biting and pulling on the straps to tighten the attachment.[2]

1 Robb et al., "Osteobiography," 18.

2 Micarelli et al., "Survival to Amputation in Pre-Antibiotic Era."

DOI: 10.17302/asgs32685 © Arc Humanities Press

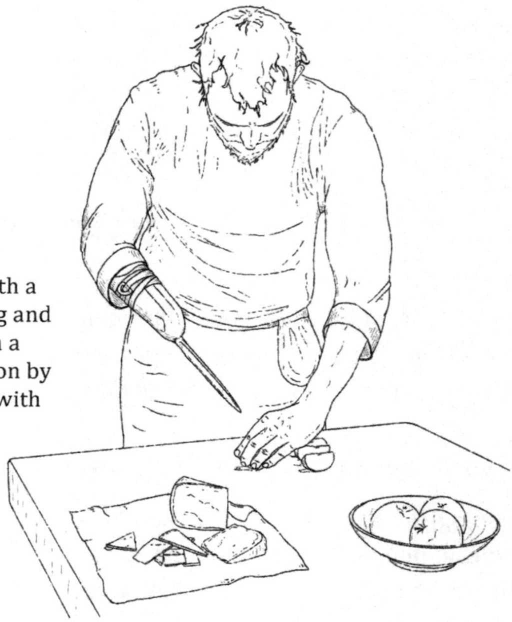

Figure 4. Drawing of a man with a knife-hand prosthetic standing and chopping vegetables, based on a Longobard skeleton. Illustration by Dayanna Knight. Reproduced with permission.

Written on Our Bodies

In a 2020 virtual talk for the Columbia University Graduate School of Architecture, Planning and Preservation entitled "The Preservation of Disability," the renowned disability studies scholar Rosemarie Garland-Thomson commented that "disability is the history of our encounters between flesh and world written on our bodies."[3] There is perhaps no more illustrative example of this statement than prosthetics.

One of the first prosthetics that we have evidence of is the Cairo Toe, which was found in a grave close to Luxor, Egypt, dating around the early first millennium BCE. The grave's occupant was a female mummy about fifty or sixty years of age and a priest's daughter; on her foot was a wooden toe.[4]

It is important to note that the amputation site was well healed. Sometimes, with medical procedures, an amputation could mean death. Scientists and archaeologists are very interested when there is evidence that certain wounds have healed over time because it means the person kept living after the procedure and they went on with their lives. We also have evidence that this particular prosthetic was refitted several times, and, in addition to a belt strap, it has mobility in the extension so the toe could balance and move a bit as the person walked.

---

3 See Columbia University Graduate School of Architecture, Planning and Preservation, "The Preservation of Disability."

4 Egyptian Museum, "Prosthetic Toe of Tabaket en Mut."

Prior to the discovery of the Cairo Toe, it was believed that the oldest example of a prosthetic was the Roman Capua Leg from 300 BCE, found next to a male skeleton missing a lower right leg. The inside was wood to about the knee; the rest of it was covered in bronze, which raises questions about the weight and comfort of wearing it. Unfortunately, like so many other pieces of cultural heritage, the Roman Capua Leg was actually destroyed in World War II during an air raid on London, but we do fortunately have a copy and another version has been 3D printed.[5]

Many of the objects mentioned are made of wood, but wood is a material that disintegrates after a while. Depending on where they were buried or in what substances they were found, quite often what remains we have left are not the actual prosthetics but the attachments, which tended to be made out of materials like iron. In the case of the Longobard man, excavators found a D-shaped buckle close to the end of his right forearm, indicating that it was used to attach the prosthesis. It is similar to other attachments that have been found, such as a circular iron ring found with a thirty-five to fifty-year-old male in Hemmaberg, Austria, dated to the sixth century.[6]

What Is a "Whole" Body?

Prosthetics are related to the human sense of body: what it is, what it "should" look like, how it "should" function." With prosthetics in particular, there is a relationship between how the body appears and how it performs. Jason Daley of the *Smithsonian Magazine* interviewed Katherine Ott, a curator of the division of medicine and science at The National Museum of American History, who spoke about the "tension between aesthetics and functionality since people first crafted artificial limbs":

> "It's always been an issue and there's never a single answer.... Every era and culture has different definition of what they consider body integrity what makes you whole." Though many of these early prostheses were likely challenging and uncomfortable to wear, "they prevent people from staring and make the user feel more integrated [into society].[7]

Missing pieces of the body raise questions of what is "normal" and what it means to have a "whole" body. To be "whole," do you need all your body parts or at least something in their place? There is a theory of the social model of disability that asserts humans are not actually disabled by physical

5 el Damaty, Hazubski, and Otte, "ArtiFacts."

6 Binder et al., "Prosthetics in Antiquity."

7 Daley, "This 3,000-Year-Old Wooden Toe."

impairments, but rather more by how society perceives that disability and does or does not accommodate it.[8] There are also issues of access. In modern terms, we can talk about insurance and whether insurance pays for certain types of prosthetics, which raises questions about who has the opportunity to think about aesthetics. What if you cannot afford a prosthetic that looks more "human" or even afford any prosthesis at all?

The Cairo Toe appears to be a both practical and cosmetic prosthetic. A practical prosthetic is one that actually helps the body do something. A cosmetic one is mainly worn for how it looks, often catering to social demands to hide "imperfections." The Cairo Toe appears to help with balance, although scientists are attempting to test that theory by making replicas and having modern people with missing toes try them out. It also, however, was developed to appear natural-looking. Another Egyptian toe prosthetic from approximately 1295–664 BCE does not bend, leading to the conclusion that it was almost exclusively cosmetic. There is also a hole for the toenail into which it is believed the wearer would put rocks or other decorations. It also has holes around the edges, as if it would have been sewn to a sock or sandal strap to keep it in place, raising questions about how comfortable or useful it would have been to wear.[9]

In addition, an eye prosthesis from 2900–2800 BCE Iran, also found with a female twenty-eight to thirty-five years old, makes us think about the sacrifices that might be made for looks. This eye, worn like a patch, was made from bitumen, animal fat, and gold wire, and it features lines and diamond patterns. While found black, researchers believe it was probably painted white to mimic an eye. However, there is evidence of abscesses, which are believed to have been caused by infection from wearing it.[10] This eye is not going to help the wearer see and is thus purely cosmetic. Why, then, would they suffer the infection in order to keep wearing it?

In the British Museum description of the second Egyptian toe, there is reference to the Cairo Toe as well as another one found with a female mummy that is now in the Albany Institute of History. While this is certainly a small sample size of female prosthetic users, it might be interesting to consider the gender of wearers of either partially or fully cosmetic prosthetics and whether women in particular might feel societal pressure to consider aesthetics, even above their own health.

---

8 See *Demystifying Disability* by Emily Ladau for discussions of various models for thinking about disability.

9 British Museum, "Cartonnage (Prosthetic Toe)."

10 Sajjadi et al., "Sistan and Baluchistan Project."

To Mimic the Human Body or Not

Another major question in prosthetics is whether to mimic the human body or not. It is widely acknowledged that what we create often cannot function as well as the human body does no matter what we do with a prosthetic. There is also an idea that, according to Katherine Ott, "[g]enerally prosthetics that mimic body parts don't work as well...They are usually clumsy and fatiguing." After World War I, Georg Schlesinger, head of the Test Center for Replacement Limbs in Berlin, "reasoned that airplanes could fly without imitating birds' wings, so why did prosthetics have to mimic arms and legs?"[11] He was by far not the first to consider such an idea.

A prosthetic leg found in China dating from approximately 300–200 BCE belonged to a biological male, fifty to sixty-five years old, whose femur and tibia had fused together, probably due to tuberculosis, which fixed the knee at an eighty-degree angle. The prosthetic included a thigh stabilizer, peg, and leather straps. Whoever created this prosthetic, however, did not mimic a human foot, but rather used an Asiatic ass (or horse) hoof, which was known for its sink resistance, thereby taking advantage of how animals walk to improve the design.[12] Today, we see athletes with prosthetics that are designed to allow them to perform, but do not necessarily look like human limbs.

Despite this evidence, we do often continue to try to mimic the human body, generally in service of the cosmetic rather than the practical. As the artist Frida Kahlo, who had a prosthetic leg painted like a red boot with Asian motifs, which is on display at the Frida Kahlo Museum, wrote to her husband, fellow artist Diego Rivera, in 1953: "They want to hurt my pride by cutting a leg off...I told you I've counted myself as incomplete for a long time, but why the fuck does everybody else need to know about it too? Now my fragmentation will be obvious for everyone to see, for you to see."[13] Kahlo's focus seems to be on others seeing her with an amputated leg and ultimately perceiving her as lacking. Given the persistent backlash against athletes with disabilities, which claims that somehow their often-non-human-shaped yet high-functioning prosthetic technology gives them an unfair advantage, it is unsurprising there is still a trend towards hiding prosthetics by matching them to their human body counterparts instead of focusing exclusively on function.[14]

---

11 Schlich, "The 'Bionic Men' of World War I."

12 Li et al., "Archaeological and Palaeopathological Study."

13 Digitized at Letters of Note.

14 See Potok, "Prosthetic Legs Don't Give Athletes Unfair Advantage."

Form and Function

Post-World War I, when many soldiers were returning with amputated limbs, inventions were devised that built prosthetics doubling as work tools. For instance:

> [the] Siemens-Schuckert-Works Universal Arm, invented in 1916, was a remarkable example of functional efficiency. It was basically a tool-holder with interchangeable parts. Its "hands" ranged from a simple hammer to cutlery with elongated handles to inserts whose ends could be attached to machines. It could serve the carpenter, farmer, draughtsman, locksmith, lathe-turner, cabinet-maker or tinsmith.[15]

The Universal Arm was basically a tool holder with interchangeable parts. It was designed to "[merge] man and machine, leaving the disabled man firmly attached to his work station. An amputee veteran would arrive at his work place in the factory, hook up the remaining part of his limb to the prosthesis, which in turn would be linked to one of the industrial machines in the factory."[16] This so-called innovation raises issues of exploitation and even, perhaps, abuse.

One function of prosthetics is to make it possible for an individual to continue participating in daily life and activities, particularly their profession. We cannot know for sure that was the case for the Longobard man, but it is indeed plausible. A famous image from a French manuscript of the *Arthurian Romances* (Yale University, Beinecke Rare Book and Manuscript Library, MS 229, fol. 257v) ca. 1290–1300, depicts a knight resting on a cane with one hand and holding a sword with the other, while his clearly amputated leg is propped on a prosthetic. Given the figure's stance and the weapon he is brandishing, he is clearly still participating in the profession that matches the garb that he is wearing. The prosthetic and the cane allow him to continue to do his job.

Immortalized by writer and poet Johann Wolfgang von Goethe, Gottfried "Götz" von Berlichingen—also called Götz of the Iron Hand—lived from 1480–1562. He owned one of the more well-known late medieval prosthetics. An imperial knight and mercenary in Germany, his right arm was amputated at the wrist during a siege at Landshut, Bavaria, when, supposedly, a cannonball pinned his arm up against his body. He ended up having two prosthetics, both of which are at Jagsthausen Castle (see Fig. 5). His first one was rudimentary, made (according to legend) by a blacksmith, out of necessity. It

15 Schlich, "The 'Bionic Men' of World War I."

16 Schlich, "The 'Bionic Men' of World War I."

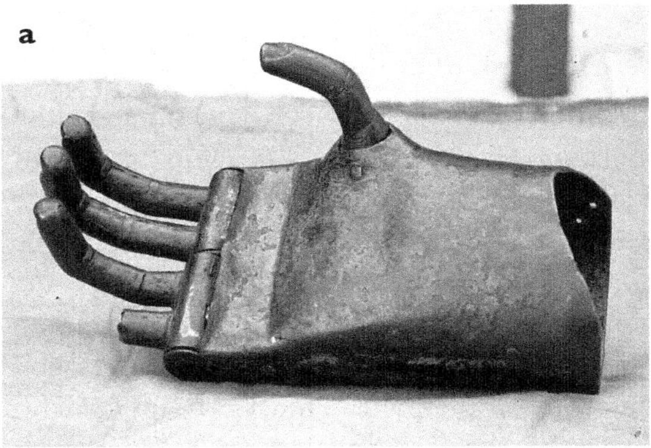

Figure 5. Two prosthetics of Götz of the Iron Hand from Jagsthausen Castle, in Landesarchiv Baden-Württemberg Generallandesarchiv Karlsruhe, Germany:

a) The right hand, item no. 498-1, no. 4108, http://www.landesarchiv-bw.de/plink/?f=4-1081855-1;
b) Forearm, item no. 498-1, no. 936, http://www.landesarchiv-bw.de/plink/?f=4-1078685.
Public domain.

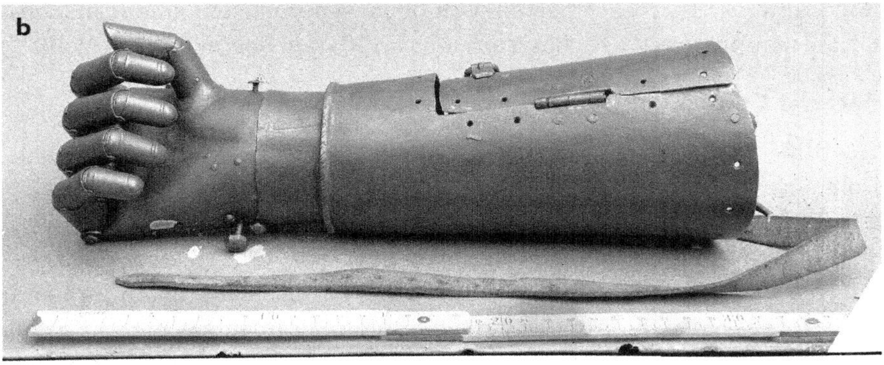

does not move, making it much more of an iron claw and cosmetic. The second one he had created has jointed fingers and is capable of holding objects. He actually could set it so that it could hold a sword or another weapon, which was more practical. Götz continued to function as a knight and mercenary for at least another forty years.[17]

These examples bring us back to the Longobard man with the knife-hand prosthetic, which certainly does not mimic a human hand. It may be that he engaged in a profession in which a knife would have been useful; thus it makes sense to fashion that into a prosthetic. We do not know if this individual used other, interchangeable devices besides a knife, but that too is not outside the realm of imagination. At any rate, we know that he used a prosthetic on a regular basis, that the use left its mark on his body, and that the knife-hand was the one that joined him in his grave.

17 Ashmore et al., "ArtiFacts."

Child with Down Syndrome

Saint-Jean-des-Vignes, France, fifth to sixth centuries

Down syndrome is a genetic condition that happens when a person has a full or partial extra copy of chromosome 21. It was named in 1866 as a result of the work of English physician John Langdon Down. While certainly its characteristics were known before that, Down was the first who clinically described the condition. It was not until 1959 that French physician Jérôme Lejeune discovered the chromosomal connection. Some of the common traits of Down syndrome are "small stature, an upward slant to the eyes, and a single deep crease across the center of the palm.... Most individuals with Down syndrome have cognitive delays that are mild to moderate." It must be noted, however, that "each person with Down syndrome is a unique individual and may possess these characteristics to different degrees, or not at all."[18]

Material Culture

According to the Centers for Disease Control and Prevention, Down syndrome occurs in about one in every 640 babies born in the United States.[19] It is difficult to calculate the historical percentages of people with Down syndrome, but it is certain that it is a condition that existed for a long time before it was officially named: "On the basis of both material culture and skeletal remains exhibiting Down syndrome like phenotypes, and basic logic, it is likely that Down syndrome has been present in mankind for as long as chromosome 21 has existed."[20] This material culture is often artistic representations of people with characteristics of Down syndrome, and researchers have found these in a number of different cultures around the world and across a long span of time periods.[21] Two of these are a Toltec terracotta figurine from approximately 500 and the sixteenth-century Flemish painting *The Adoration of the Christ Child* (in the New York Metropolitan Museum of Art collection).

The Toltecs lived in Mexico, flourishing especially from 950–1150. Maria Luisa Martinez-Frias identified a terracotta figurine of a head with Down syndrome characteristics, including short palpebral fissures, oblique eyes, midfacial hypoplasia, an open mouth, and a protruding tongue.[22] John M.

---

18 National Down Syndrome Society, "About Down Syndrome."

19 Centers for Disease Control and Prevention, "Living with Down Syndrome."

20 Starbuck, "On the Antiquity of Trisomy 21," 33.

21 See Starbuck, "On the Antiquity of Trisomy 21."

22 Martinez-Frias, "The Real Earliest Historical Evidence of Down Syndrome," 231.

Starbuck classified this figurine as "arguably one of the highest quality depictions of Down syndrome in material culture."[23]

In 2003, Andrew S. Levitas and Cheryl S. Reid analyzed *The Adoration of the Christ Child* (painted around 1515), focusing on an angel on Mary's left as well as a shepherd above the centre angel.[24] They conclude that both have characteristics of Down syndrome. The angel has a "flattened midface, epicanthic folds, upslanted palpebral fissures, small and upturned nasal tip, downward curving mouth corners, and short fingers with a widely spaced and curving small finger," and the shepherd "is portrayed with a similar facial composition; however, the upslanted palpebral fissures are slightly longer and this individual has widely spaced eyes."[25] Starbuck also notes that angel figures in the upper left of the painting have similar characteristics. He points out that there is another nearly identical version of *The Adoration of the Christ Child* painted around the same time, which does not give these features to these individuals. Levitas and Reid discuss the possible implications for disability of depicting an angel with Down syndrome and suggest "one of the following: individuals with disabilities were portrayed for symbolic purposes, the artist had warm feelings towards the models who had disabilities, or the physical signs of Down syndrome were not recognized at the time of this painting as a predictor of disability."[26] Other paintings have also been examined with this lens: *The Virgin and Child* by Andrea Mantegna (1463–1465), *The Madonna and Child* also by Andrea Mantegna (1431–1506), and *The Adoration of the Shepherds* by Jacob Jordaen (1650).

Given past beliefs that Down syndrome is a modern disease, identifying historical artistic representations of individuals with these characteristics is essential in recognizing the long heritage of the condition and the place of people with Down syndrome in our human story.

A Child in France

At the Abbey of Saint-Jean-des-Vignes in northeastern France, in 1989, archaeologists discovered almost one hundred skeletons from a fifth- to sixth-century burial site. In studies in 1994 and 2009, researchers suggested the possibility that one of these, a five to seven-year-old child, might have had Down syndrome. In 2014, Maïté Rivollat et al. completed an extensive

23 Starbuck, "On the Antiquity of Trisomy 21," 31.

24 Levitas and Reid, "An Angel with Down Syndrome."

25 Starbuck, "On the Antiquity of Trisomy 21," 28.

26 Starbuck, "On the Antiquity of Trisomy 21," 28.

study on the skull of this child.[27] In comparing this skull with others of children in the same age range from a similar time period as well as modern children, they noted "a large cephalicindex, a flat occipital bone, less obtuse values of vault curvature angles, dental agenesis, periodontitis, thinness of cranial vault, ametopic suture and lambdoid wormian bones," among other characteristics.[28] Given this, they confirm the diagnosis of the child having Down syndrome. Potentially, this child is the earliest and youngest case to be identified with a degree of certainty.

Tracing a Disability through Multiple Sources

Evidence for the historical presence of a disability such as Down syndrome is stronger when different types of sources are examined together. Here, we have artistic and osteological evidence to help frame the story of this condition. Other disabilities can also be tracked in this way. Arthrogryposis Multiplex Congenita is, according to the National Organization for Rare Disorders, "a group of congenital (present at birth) conditions characterized by joint contractures in two or more joints of the body."[29] The skeleton of a thirty-five to forty-five-year old early medieval male, uncovered at Saint Gregory's Priory in Canterbury, England, "show[s] a combination of abnormalities that are highly suggestive" of this disorder, including a fused club foot.[30] Simultaneously, the twelfth century *The Life and Miracles of St William of Norwich* by Thomas of Monmouth describes an eight-year-old girl named Agnes:

> She could not raise herself, nor could she at any time turn from one side to the other without assistance. In addition, to make things worse, because the sinews in her neck had contracted, her left cheek adhered to her left shoulder so closely that one was embedded in the other. Moreover, her neck could not be bent in any direction whatever without bending her shoulder.[31]

Eleanora C. Gordon has interpreted these conditions as a description of Arthrogryposis Multiplex Congenita, providing a literary source to support the archaeological one.[32]

27 Rivollat et al., "Ancient Down Syndrome."

28 Rivollat et al., "Ancient Down Syndrome," 13.

29 National Organization for Rare Disorders, "Arthrogryposis Multiplex Congenita."

30 Anderson and Thomas, "A Possible Case," 181.

31 Translation provided by Gordon, "Arthrogryposis Multiplex Congenita," 80.

32 Thank you to Maria Johnson for bringing these two sources to my attention.

Reading a Burial

The 2014 study of the child at the Abbey of Saint-Jean-des-Vignes revealed further insights into the life of the child with Down syndrome. The researchers suggested that "this Down syndrome child was not treated differently at death than others in the community. We interpret this as meaning that the child was maybe not stigmatized during life, the first time a Down syndrome individual has been so viewed in the context of the ancient community."[33] This interpretation is significant in thinking about the experience of people with disabilities and of those with Down syndrome in particular. In this context and community, this child does not seem to have been treated differently.

Certainly, such an example does not speak to the experience of every person. We do have potential evidence in other circumstances of the burials of people with disabilities indicating some level of stigma. An individual known as the Coppergate Woman found in York, England, between 1976 and 1981 and then studied in 2010, revealed a late ninth-century female with hip dysplasia, with

> disuse and wasting of the affected leg and hip, over-use of the opposite leg causing muscular trauma and osteoarthritis and one-sided degenerative joint disease and osteoarthritis of the spine...may have used crutches and had unusually robust arms and shoulders, as well as degenerative joint disease in the shoulders, hips and right hand.[34]

Her skeleton was found at a distance from the other bodies discovered at the same time, and it is possible that this difference in burial location, especially as no other burials have been located in that area, indicates potential ostracism.[35]

We also have examples of people with disabilities being buried in places of honour. A male body approximately thirty years old, who lived between 1300 and 1536, was found with thousands of others from 1982 to 1984 at the Trinitatis cemetery in Lund, Scania. He had severe fractures of the left knee, which "healed at a 45-degree angulation" and "was fused at the time of trauma."[36] The body was "buried on top of the foundation stones at the base of the western church tower" and "proximity to the church, and his burial

33 Rivollat et al., "Ancient Down Syndrome," 14.

34 Holst, "Osteological Analysis Coppergate York," iv.

35 JORVIK Viking Centre, "The People of JORVIK."

36 Nolan et al., "Disability and Care in Late Medieval Lund," 9.

atop the foundation stones of the church's western tower, indicates a position of upper socioeconomic status" implying that the individual's "status within society was not wholly defined by disability."[37]

Reading burials provides a significant amount of information related to the perception of those with disabilities, but collectively they reinforce that these perceptions are related to individual circumstances and cannot be generalized to everyone.

STORIES: Finding Richard III, the Scoliotic King

Leicester Cathedral, England, fifteenth century

King of England from 1483 to 1485, Richard III is both a well-known example of disability heritage as well as archaeological discoveries. After Richard was killed, historically marking the end of his dynastic line, his body mysteriously disappeared. Researchers later found evidence that suggested he could have been buried at what was previously Grey Friars Church, which had been turned into a car park near Leicester Cathedral. The chances of being able to locate the actual body were very low, making the discovery in 2012 rather astonishing.

Identifying the skeleton as the king's took quite a bit of work. When the skeleton was uncovered, further study of the teeth and skull as well as the presence of a Y-chromosome determined he was a male in his thirties. Richard was thirty-two when he died. He is known to have been killed in the Battle of Bosworth Field in the Wars of the Roses, making wounds likely, and the skeleton's wounds were identified as being made prior to death by weapons of the medieval period. He likely had a high-status diet, supported by the chemical elements in his bones. The circumstantial but scientific evidence mounted up. More definitive evidence came later through DNA testing. The researchers tracked down two living descendants of Richard's sister, finding that their mitochondrial DNA was a match.

As the leader of the verification team, Turi King has confirmed, statistically, there is a 99.999% certainty that the skeleton they found is Richard III, ensuring that the correct body was reinterred in Leicester Cathedral in 2015 (see Fig. 6).[38] While important as an historical find, the identification of Richard also contributed to disability heritage.

---

37 Nolan et al., "Disability and Care in Late Medieval Lund," 6, 13.

38 King, "We Proved, with 99.999% Certainty, That the Skeleton in the Car Park was Richard III."

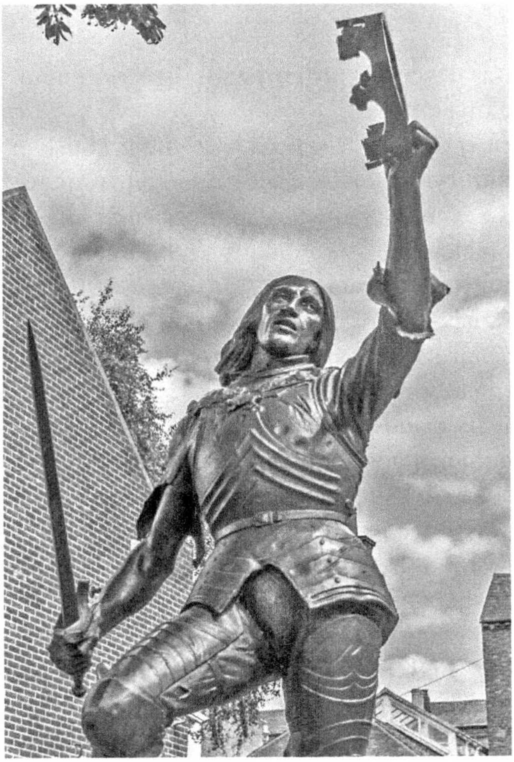

Figure 6. Richard III statue, Leicester Cathedral. Leicester, England. Photograph by author.

The skeleton displayed a distinctive characteristic that helped to pinpoint his identity: a curved spine. The famous description of a hunchbacked Richard by William Shakespeare in his *Richard III* is more a product of anti-Plantagenet propaganda than reality. I discuss Shakespeare's contribution to the image of Richard in *Why Study the Middle Ages?*:

> Sir Thomas More, a staunch advocate of the Tudors, wrote *The History of Richard III* around 1513–1518, approximately thirty years after Richard's death. The *History*, which does not present Richard in a positive light, places a significant emphasis on the king's physical appearance, implying a connection between that and his apparently flawed character.... More's work was one of the primary sources for Shakespeare's *Richard III* in which the king, depicted as a malicious character, is called a "bunchback'd toad" (Act I, Scene 3). The character of Richard himself, in his first speech opening the play, describes his various physical characteristics as "deformed, unfinish'd," directly linking his disability and what he defines as his resulting deficiencies with his decision to "prove a villain" (Act I, Scene 1). Much has been written about the productions of the play that visually make this link with Richard's hunchback overemphasized. It is Shakespeare's representation that has survived to modern day, reinforcing the persistent image of the "evil disabled."[39]

Although the extreme depiction of Richard is an invention, there are more contemporary descriptions that indicate the king did have a spinal irregularity that was likely a result of scoliosis. For instance, chronicler and author

39 Tracy, *Why Study the Middle Ages?*, 59–60.

of *Historia Regum Angliae* John Rous describes Richard with "unequal shoulders, the right higher and the left lower."[40]

Greek physician and philosopher Galen is credited with the first use of the term *scoliosis* in the second century. Scoliosis is, according to the American Association of Neurological Surgeons (AANS), "an abnormal lateral curvature of the spine." The National Scoliosis Foundation (NSF) defines it as a lateral deviation that is greater than ten degrees. Today, they estimate that scoliosis affects approximately 2–3% of the population, with higher instances in women. Studies of Richard's body suggest that his was "adolescent onset idiopathic scoliosis, probably starting after 10 years of age."[41]

AANS outlines potential signs of scoliosis as uneven shoulders (which matches Rous's description), shoulder blades sticking out, head off centre from the pelvis, raised hips, uneven rib cage or waist, and leaning to one side. Those with idiopathic scoliosis are more likely to experience back pain. NSF notes that these symptoms can "impact the quality of life with limited activity, pain, reduced respiratory function, or diminished self-esteem." Researchers believe that Richard's scoliosis was not severe: "His trunk would have been short relative to the length of his limbs, and his right shoulder a little higher than the left…we identified no evidence that Richard would have walked with an overt limp, because the leg bones are symmetric and well formed."[42] Given that contemporaries commented on the shape of his body, we can at least surmise that it was visible to a certain extent.

The Greek physician Hippocrates developed some of the first treatments for the condition, which included "body traction and local pressure applied to the apex of the deformity," and, in the eleventh century, Persian physician Avicenna also recommended "stretching, pressure, or traction to correct bone and joint deformities."[43] Some researchers have speculated what kind of treatment Richard might have undergone for his scoliosis, particularly given his high social status. Mary Ann Lund theorizes that he could have been treated with traction, perhaps rope tied around the body and tightened to stretch the spine.[44] His high-status diet might actually have also been therapeutic. However, we cannot learn about any particular method of treatment from his skeleton.

---

40 Hanham, *Richard III and His Early Historians*, 120–21.

41 Appleby et al., "The Scoliosis of Richard III," 1944.

42 Appleby et al., "The Scoliosis of Richard III," 1944.

43 Yağcı and Bek, "A Historical Perspective of the Management of Scoliosis," 440.

44 Bryner, "Painful Treatment Possible for King Richard III's Scoliosis."

To tell the story of Richard III's body has involved a number of disciplines working together, such as archaeology, osteobiography, palaeoproteomics, history, literature, art, genetics, forensics, statistics, and genealogy, among others. Identification of a five-hundred-year-old skeleton found under a car park requires a significant amount of investigation, but the presence of disability adds a further dimension of interdisciplinarity. NSF declares that scoliosis is a "multifactorial disorder, which requires multidisciplinary research and treatment," and studying it as a medieval disability even more so.

Section 2: Disfigurement

In *Living with Disfigurement in Early Medieval Europe*, Patricia Skinner writes that a "damaged face arguably did not bring the same levels of impairment as a serious injury to body or limb...but the social disability associated with the disruption of the facial features was potentially much greater."[45] She defines disfigurement as "an injury to the visage or surface, potentially limiting the ability to be expressive or be recognized, rather than to the social being to whom it belongs."[46] Unless it is extreme and affects a specific body part, such as the eyes, disfigurement does not generally change the physical abilities of an individual, yet can be disabling based upon the reactions of others and how the individual is treated. In her study, Skinner notes that, in cases where disfigurement is stigmatized, "ridicule" is the most prevalent reaction and fear that one's appearance will be laughed at or dismissed.[47]

Rosemarie Garland-Thomson in a study of staring discusses how seeing people with disabilities invokes "fascinated disbelief and uneasy identification [as the]...visibly disabled body intrudes on our routine visual landscape and compels our attention, often obscuring the personhood of its bearer."[48] She also comments that humans sense that an "atypical face is a failed face, perhaps an improperly human, irrationally organized face," and thus she indicates that perceptions of disfigurement can even raise questions about a person's very "humanness."[49] Further, Garland-Thomson notes that an observer can associate an "atypical face" with those of different races than their own, thereby also indicating that members of another race can be perceived as disfigured, and possibly inhuman, simply for appearing different.

---

45 Skinner, *Living with Disfigurement*, 58.

46 Skinner, *Living with Disfigurement*, 45.

47 Skinner, *Living with Disfigurement*, 160.

48 Garland-Thomson, *Staring*, 20.

49 Garland-Thomson, *Staring*, 104.

Disfigurement is the body telling a person's story. Disfigurement—or the perception of disfigurement—can be a social disability, and we can learn from how such individuals, real or fictional, are read or represented.

Scrofulous Sogolon

Female figure, terracotta with ochre/red slip, 37.6 cm (14.8 inches) tall; Inland Niger Delta region, Mali, thirteenth to fifteenth centuries; Musée du quai Branly-Jacques Chirac, Paris

The Scrofulous Sogolon refers to a collection of Djenné archaeological objects: terracotta figures dating from the thirteenth to the seventeenth centuries. Their origins and meaning remain a bit mysterious, but researchers Anne-Marie Bouttiaux and Marc Ghysels have postulated that they are related to the semi-legendary character of Sogolon: the mother of the first Emperor of Mali, Sundiata Keita. The specific object referenced here, referred to by Bouttiaux and Ghysels as MQB (given it is owned by the Musée du quai Branly-Jacques Chirac in Paris), represents many of the characteristics that are specific to these figures:

> On the torso of the MQB sculpture is a "keeled breast" (pectus carinatum), a deformity of the rib cage that forces the sternum forward in a sharp ridge like the keel of a boat. This deformity, here accentuated by several concentric tapering incisions, generally results from the fusion of costal cartilage during childhood and is commonly called "pigeon chest"...the head turned to the left, snake-shaped tears, incised nasolabial grooves, parted lips, a snake-shaped ring around the neck, an ellipsoidal dorsal hump at the top of the backbone, apparently young breasts, snakes decorating the body, and a good weight status.[50]

This description illustrates the reason for the "scrofulous"—meaning tainted, diseased, but also a reference to a specific type of tuberculosis—designation with attributes typically categorized as deformities, such as a "keeled breast," "pigeon chest," and a hunchback. To discover the connection to Sogolon, we need to turn to the *Epic of Sundiata.*

Disability in the *Epic of Sundiata*

The Malian *Epic of Sundiata* has been transmitted through oral tradition since the thirteenth century. It recounts the legendary story of Sundiata Keita, starting before his birth and continuing through to his rule. The first

50 Bouttiaux and Ghysels, "Scrofulous Sogolon," 95.

six chapters of the text (as presented by D. T. Niane) recount his mother and father meeting, his conception, and then the details of his childhood. They also illustrate several representations of disability. As Magnus Mfoafo-M'Carthy, Jeff Grischow, and Festus Moasun note, "One of the earliest written sources containing evidence of physical disability in Africa is an epic poem written about Sundiata Keita."[51]

Analyzing disability is both about recognizing the physical or mental reality of the individual as well as their social reality, i.e., how others react to the disability and how they perceive it. Sundiata, prophesied to be a great king, is represented as having "a slow and difficult childhood," for "at the age of three he still crawled along on all-fours while children of the same age were already walking."[52] We see how others react to him; in particular, his father's first wife, Sassouma Bérété. Jealous of the potential replacement of her own son, she is reported as saying to her son in front of Sundiata: "Come, my son, walk, jump, leap about. The jinn didn't promise you anything out of the ordinary, but I prefer a son who walks on his two legs to a lion that crawls on the ground."[53] She also spreads the gossip that "people had seen one-eyed kings, one-armed kings, and lame kings, but a stiff-legged king had never been heard tell of."[54] It is important to note that it is a relative villain who makes this statement, calling into question the sentiment expressed about disability. Mfoafo-M'Carthy, Grischow, and Moasun have found that "individuals with disabilities [in precolonial Africa] were considered full members of society, complete with all the responsibilities prescribed by gender, status, and age," which corroborates Sassouma's statements about the validity of kings with other types of disabilities.[55]

Eventually, at the end of this section of the epic, Sundiata forces himself to walk, the description of which is very physical and visceral. A parallel text from medieval Europe might be Bishop Asser's biography of Alfred the Great, credited with uniting England rather like Sundiata with Mali, and its description of the king's experience with what we would today call Crohn's Disease.

---

51 Mfoafo-M'Carthy, Grischow, and Moasun, *Experiencing Disability Stigma in Ghana*, 17.

52 Niane, *Sundiata*, 15. D. T. Niane's version is the first translation of the epic into English.

53 Niane, *Sundiata*, 16.

54 Niane, *Sundiata*, 18.

55 Mfoafo-M'Carthy, Grischow, and Moasun, *Experiencing Disability Stigma in Ghana*, 22.

The Disfigurement of Sogolon

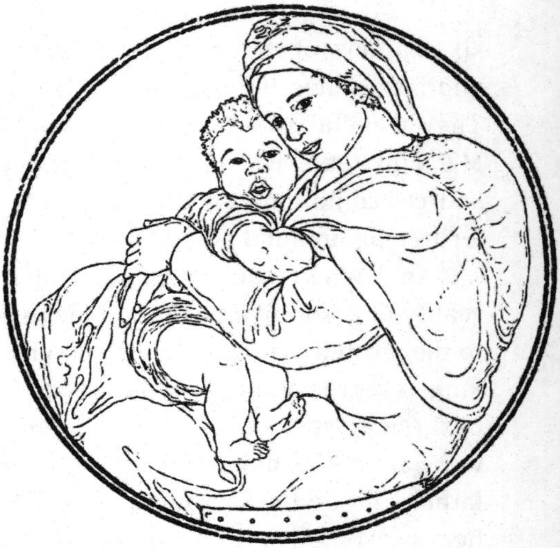

Figure 7. Sogolon Condé. Illustration by Dayanna Knight. Reproduced with permission.

Sundiata's mother, Sogolon Condé, is introduced in the *Epic* as "ugly in a sturdy sort of way" and "hideous" with "a hump which deformed her shoulders and back," "muscular arms," and "bulging breasts" (see Fig. 7 for an artistic representation).[56] Later, she is described as "a very ugly maid—uglier than you can imagine."[57] In some versions of the *Epic*, her deformities are far more extensive: in addition to being hunchbacked and ugly, she is also bald and knock-kneed with damaged eyes or tear ducts. These are ascribed to childhood injuries caused by interactions with supernatural objects when she was still too young for them.[58] When she is chosen by a pair of hunters as a reward for killing a rampaging buffalo in her home kingdom, they are ridiculed: "the king could not help laughing, and then general laughter broke out and the people split their sides with mirth."[59] The implication here is that Sogolon's features, which mark her as both disfigured and deformed, are a source of social rejection. Skinner does note a gendered aspect to disfigurement in that "women's faces were targeted as a means of marginalizing them and taking them out of the social arena."[60]

Sogolon's physical features are a primary motivator for her introduction in the *Epic*. It is foretold to the king that, if he marries a woman with her characteristics, she will bear him a son who will rule a united Mali. When she is brought before the king, it is her unique appearance that marks her as the prophesied individual. Unfortunately, fulfilling prophecy comes with a tragic price. After the king makes her his second wife, the text describes how Sogolon is able to prevent him from consummating the relationship by fighting his wraith, or spirit, with her own. She is successful, emphasizing

56 Niane, *Sundiata*, 6–7.

57 Niane, *Sundiata*, 8

58 Conrad, *Sunjata*, 42–43.

59 Niane, *Sundiata*, 9.

60 Skinner, *Living with Disfigurement*, 150.

her strength, until he claims he has been told by supernatural beings that she must die. In a fright, she faints, preventing her wraith from being able to protect her. The king rapes and impregnates her while she is unconscious.

Sogolon is depicted even before her physical introduction in the text as "an extraordinary woman" in spite of possessing what are described as "ugly" features and a hunchback.[61] Distinguished historian of medieval Africa David Conrad remarks in his translation of the epic with Djanka Tassey Condé's narration that Tassey Condé specifically notes, "A source of greatness will not be acquired without hardship"—a common feature among stories of epic heroes.[62] Sogolon maintains a significant position in her son's life, exemplifying many of the functions often exhibited by African queen-mothers. As Tarikhu Farrar comments, "Female title-holders placed in the highest levels of the political order were a common feature of ancient and later pre-colonial African political systems."[63] In her own right, Sogolon is powerful: a healer, a sorceress, a survivor, a diplomat. Indeed, Sundiata takes his name from her, rather than his father, King Naré Maghan. Her healing abilities are well-renowned and are made all the more formidable by the exception when she fails to heal her son's deformed legs when he is a child: "Her son's infirmity weighed heavily upon Sogolon Kedjou; she had resorted to all her talent as a sorceress to give strength to her son's legs but the rarest herbs had been useless."[64] Sogolon is pronounced "a wise mother."[65] This wisdom takes many forms. She manages her son's safe exile when his half-brother succeeds their father, leading him through many lands and securing allies for him through her diplomacy. Despite finding comfortable circumstances among these allies, Sogolon does not let Sundiata forget his true destiny:

> Sogolon knew that the time had arrived and she had performed her task. She had nurtured the son for whom the world was waiting and she knew that now her mission was accomplished, while that of Djata [Sundiata] was about to begin. One day she said to her son, "Do not deceive yourself. Your destiny lies not here but in Mali. The moment has come. I have finished my task and it is yours that is going to begin, my son. But you must be able to wait. Everything in its own good time."[66]

---

61 Niane, *Sundiata*, 11.

62 Conrad, *Sunjata*, xxi.

63 Farrar, "The Queenmother, Matriarchy, and the Question," 579.

64 Niane, *Sundiata*, 16.

65 Niane, *Sundiata*, 26.

66 Niane, *Sundiata*, 37–38.

In this quotation, we have a succinct summary of Sogolon's interpretation—bound up in the word "nurtured"—of her role as a queen-mother, of a mother to the prophesized *mansa*. In essence, she enables the creation of the empire of Mali. She is contrasted with her co-wife, Sassouma Bérété, who, due to a similar if distorted interpretation of her role, persecutes Sogolon and Sundiata out of fear for her own son's title inheritance.

After Sogolon marries the king, her physical characteristics cease to be a concern. They are rarely mentioned and no longer determine the reaction of others to her. Her disfigurement seems to serve the purpose of marking her as significant and of underscoring that appearance does not dictate destiny.

Sogolon's Influence

The character of Sogolon has had a lasting influence. She regularly appears in plays, songs, and fiction even in the modern day, and no retelling of Sundiata Keita is complete without her presence. Conrad dubs her "one of the greatest heroines of Manding oral tradition."[67] Bouttiaux and Ghysels emphasize this fame in addition to the characteristics attributed to her in various versions of the epic as evidence for identifying the Scrofulous Sogolon terracotta figures with her, stating that they "seem consistent with some of the stigmata... especially the hunched, or gibbous, back; the protuberant eyes running with tears (shown as snakes); and the obvious ugliness."[68] These figures are, like Sogolon herself, distinctive for their deformities and disfigurement, reminding us that such characteristics create unique art and stories.

Goddess Cōātlīcue Statue

Andesite, 2.5 m (8.3 feet) tall; Aztec, 1439 or 1491; Museo Nacional de Antropología, Mexico City

The statue of Cōātlīcue represents the Aztec goddess who gave birth to the moon and stars. Possibly completed between 1439 to 1491, it was buried in Tenochtitlan after the 1521 Spanish conquest and then excavated in 1790 only to be reinterred. It was then excavated again in 1803, reburied, and finally unearthed for good in 1823.

Imposing at over eight-feet tall, the statue is a complex combination of imagery. Cōātlīcue's head displays two snakes rising out of her neck and facing each other while her neck has a line of circles indicating decapitation.

---

67 Conrad, *Sunjata*, xxi.

68 Bouttiaux and Ghysels, "Scrofulous Sogolon," 97.

Likewise, her hands are snakes, possibly also indicating dismemberment. Her sagging breasts indicate she has given birth and are covered by a necklace of human hearts and hands. She has a skirt made of snakes, representing her name, which translates to "Snakes-Her-Skirt."

The Myths of Cōātlīcue

Like most myths, there are many versions of Cōātlīcue's stories, not the least in this case because most of them have been sifted through colonial filters, such as Franciscan Bernardino de Sahagún, who wrote down the Nahuatl *Florentine Codex* in the sixteenth century. One of the most famous of Cōātlīcue's stories is the birth of her son Huītzilōpōchtli, the god of sun and war and patron god of the Aztecs. While carrying him, one of her daughters, Coyolxāuhqui, becomes upset about the pregnancy, considering the miraculous conception dishonourable. Coyolxāuhqui leads her four hundred brothers against their mother, but Huītzilōpōchtli bursts forth, fully grown and armed. He decapitates his sister, defeats the other brothers, and protects his mother. In some versions, he places Coyolxāuhqui in the sky as the moon. This story is less about Cōātlīcue than it is about her son, yet it has been the main focus in attempts to decipher the Cōātlīcue statue.[69]

Cecelia F. Klein offers a different perspective. In trying to explain features of the statue that do not reflect the Huītzilōpōchtli story (such as it is her daughter, not her, who is decapitated), Klein postulates that Cōātlīcue is one of five female deities who are said to have sacrificed themselves in order either to create the current sun or to make it move. While various names for these women appear in different texts, the *Historia de los mexicanos por sus pinturas*—a Spanish codex written in the 1530s possibly by Franciscan Andrés de Olmos—names Cōātlīcue as one of the "group of heroic women whose collective death not only enabled the creation and survival of the universe, but the government as well."[70] Thus, "Coatlicue sacrificed herself voluntarily to provide the Mexica with the warmth, light, and changing seasons that brought them crops, food, and good health."[71] Recentring the focus of the statue on this story elevates the goddess as a hero of humankind in her own right rather than as only the mother of one.

The most compelling evidence for this interpretation is the statue's snake skirt. Not only a representation of the translation of Cōātlīcue's name,

69 Klein, "A New Interpretation of the Aztec Statue," 231.

70 Klein, "A New Interpretation of the Aztec Statue," 243.

71 Klein, "A New Interpretation of the Aztec Statue," 245.

it also plays an important role in the sun myth. The five women who sacrificed themselves left their skirts behind as a form of memento of their deed; afterwards, they were kept as relics. Legend then indicates that the women were resurrected either by or literally transformed into these skirts, thereby imbuing their identities into them. The skirt on the Cōātlīcue statue is one of its prominent features, creating perhaps even a secondary relic that petitioners could seek out for aid, especially given it is believed the statue was originally displayed at a prominent temple, the *Templo Mayor*.[72] Coupling the skirt with the signs of sacrifice in the decapitation and dismemberment imagery creates a powerful visual of Cōātlīcue's story.

Disfiguring Misinterpretations

The disfigurement of the Cōātlīcue statue came later in its history. It begins when the statue is "discovered" and unearthed in 1790, or rather the story continues when we consider the initial need during the Spanish conquest to hide the statue for fear of it being destroyed. Its founding was an accident, a side effect of the construction of an underground aqueduct. Moved to the Real y Pontificia Universidad de México, it soon found itself reburied by Catholic clergymen, likely out of concern it could reignite indigenous religions but ostensibly because they did not want "Mexican youth to be exposed to such a horrible sight."[73] Here begins the tradition of the statue being read "through European aesthetics," "as an object of curiosity and horror instead of as an abstract sculpture that narrated through its body the foundation of the Aztec empire."[74] To the Aztec people, it is representative of their cultural story. To the Europeans, it was evidence that the Aztec people were indeed "barbaric" and "uncivilized."

The next time the Cōātlīcue statue makes an appearance is in 1803, when the Prussian scientist Alexander von Humboldt had it unearthed once again for a brief time. In his *Vues des cordillères, et monuments des peuples indigenes de l'Amérique* (1810), he does manage to appreciate the craftsmanship of the statue, but, beyond that, he clearly sees it as repugnant. As Ann De León states:

> The Aztecs become barbaric because of their "incorrect" esthetics. For Humboldt, Coatlicue's body performs an "incorrect" esthetics because it does not present a mimetic or naturalistic representation of the female human body.

72 Klein, "A New Interpretation of the Aztec Statue," 244.

73 De León, "Coatlicue," 260.

74 De León, "Coatlicue," 260.

> By incorporating human and non-human parts what is created is a monstrous body.[75]

Indeed, Humboldt concludes that the Cōātlīcue statue must depict death because it "did not constitute a realistic and anatomically faithful representation of a woman" and "the visible mutilated body parts and organs can only mean a dead body."[76] What Humboldt saw was a disfigured, and thus repellant, female body, and, when he was done studying the statue, it was buried away back in the ground.

Human Exhibitions

The disabling of the Cōātlīcue statue did not end with Humboldt. In 1823, the English antiquarian William Bullock arrived in Mexico with an interest in the statue and secured its final release from the ground. Bullock's intention was to open the first exhibition of Mexican antiquities in London at the Egyptian Hall in Piccadilly, for which he was loaned over fifty artifacts from the Mexican government and created a life-size plaster cast reproduction of the Cōātlīcue statue. This exhibition was less educational than it was a "theatre of horrors and freak-show cabinet of curiosities," including among its "virtual-reality-like exhibit" a "living human being," Jose Cayetana Ponce de Leon from the village of Chyula, a "noble savage."[77] This exhibition served "part of the British Empire's goal of capturing foreign material culture to aggrandize its empire and to capture and display the subjugated 'other.'"[78] Bullock himself identifies Cōātlīcue not as a goddess or as a part of Aztec heritage but rather as "a monstrous representative of deformity and carnage" that would delight his audience with its horror.[79] As Garland-Thomson notes, the fascination or repulsion someone might feel at viewing disability can overshadow the humanity of the person being viewed. In the case of the Cōātlīcue statue, it overshadowed the cultural significance of the artifact and the story it has to tell.

Human exhibitions such as Bullock's are unfortunately not unusual. Among his other atrocities, besides invading the Aztec empire in the sixteenth century, Hernán Cortés also assembled his own human exhibition to

---

75 De León, "Coatlicue," 266.

76 De León, "Coatlicue," 270.

77 De León, "Coatlicue," 272–75.

78 De León, "Coatlicue," 271.

79 De León, "Coatlicue," 273.

take back to Spain with him with what historian Francisco López de Gómara described as "certain Indian men and women who were very white, and others who were dwarfs, and others hunchbacks" as "a demonstration of the marvels of New Spain."[80] In his own writings, Cortés seems to justify doing so with his observations of people with disabilities in Moctezuma's court, which he perceives as objects in confinement and on display.[81]

What became known as "freak shows" mostly in North America in the late nineteenth century[82] started as "cabinets of curiosities" in Europe in the mid-sixteenth century, which developed especially in response to colonial exploration and contact with the unfamiliar. While these could resemble modern museums with collections of natural and cultural artifacts, they also could be locations for "keeping human monsters—both living and mortal remains—as a part of a collection, the purpose of which was to enhance the majesty of its owner."[83] Barbora Půtová ascribes the popularity of "freak shows" and the desire to gaze on "monstrosities" directly to colonial expansion, and she connects the perceptions of people with disabilities to those of non-European peoples: "An exotic picture of the members of non-European cultures or physically handicapped people evoked the triumph of Western civilization over technological backwardness of preliterate societies."[84] These spaces were not ones of cultural sharing and appreciation, but rather ones that reinforced perceived hierarchies and exploitation.

The inclination to view the unique and different as in some way disfigured is deeply entrenched. Even in Klein's article that reinterprets the Cōātlīcue statue, she describes the two snakes on the statue's face as "creat[ing] a monstrous head."[85] Scholars are also beginning to explore and call out the lasting disabling effects of colonialism. In the introduction to a special issue of *Postcolonial Studies* on "Disability and Postcolonialism," Esme Cleall identifies "the human body as a productive site of contest within the colonial social order, both in the attempt to impose Western modernity on the bodies of colonized people and in the imprinting of colonial ideology

80 Bearden, *Monstrous Kinds*, 127 and 131.

81 The reality of disability in the Aztec empire and in Moctezuma's court is far more complex. See Bearden, *Monstrous Kinds*, 109–41.

82 The Oxford English Dictionary records the first use of "freaks" in this context in 1883.

83 Bearden, *Monstrous Kinds*, 132.

84 Půtová, "Freak Shows," 91.

85 Klein, "A New Interpretation of the Aztec Statue," 231.

upon indigenous consciousness."[86] Within his article in the volume, Subhadeep Ray describes

> the historical fact that the colonized body and soul were never "free of internal tensions or structures of oppression" and there was no possibility of unearthing any pure "indigenism," which was continuously affected by a long and complicated process of cultural transitions set into motion by the imperial rule.[87]

The disfigurement of the Cōātlīcue statue by Humboldt and other Europeans provides a dramatic allegory of this disabling effect of colonial ideology, even to the point of dubbing indigeneity itself as a curiosity to be put on display.

Today, the Cōātlīcue statue resides in a place of honour at the Museo Nacional de Antropología in Mexico City, reclaiming, as Ann De León remarks, its rightfully "prominent place in Mexico's national and visual discourse."[88]

STORIES: Imagining Egil Skallagrímsson's Legendary Skull

Narrative Descriptions from Egil's Saga, Iceland, Thirteenth Century

The figure of warrior and poet Egil (also spelled Egill) Skallagrímsson is deeply embedded in Icelandic heritage. What is known about him comes from *Egil's Saga*, the earliest manuscript of which dates to around 1250 and details events from 870–1030. Like most of the sagas, it follows the history of Egil's family, both those who came before and after him, starting with his grandfather.

Within the saga, Egil is described as a massive, imposing figure with distinct features:

> Egil was large-featured, broad of forehead, with large eyebrows, a nose not long but very thick, lips wide and long, chin exceeding broad, as was all about the jaws; thick-necked was he, and big-shouldered beyond other men, hard-featured, and grim when angry. He was well-made, more than commonly tall, had hair wolf-gray and thick, but became early bald. He was black-eyed and brown-skinned. (Ch. 55)[89]

---

86 Cleall, "Disability and Postcolonialism," 6.

87 Ray, "Dialectics of Impairment," 119.

88 De León, "Coatlicue," 260.

89 All references to *Egil's Saga* are provided with the chapter number and quoted from: "Egils Saga," *wikisaga*. https://wikisaga.hi.is/index.php?title=Category:Egils_saga._Efnisyfirlit.

Taken as a whole, these characteristics make a startling impression: large head, thick nose and lips, broad chin. Well-known for his way with words, Egil refers to himself on numerous occasions as ugly; in Chapter 63, he jokingly says his "features [are] loathly." Scholar Jesse Byock remarks that it would be "highly unusual for the physical features of a saga protagonist to be portrayed in so grotesque a manner, unless the writer was reporting a well-known story."[90] Byock also reminds us that these characteristics run in Egil's family: "Egill resembles his father and grandfather; both are remembered in the saga as physically menacing and physiologically different from their otherwise fair and handsome kinsmen."[91] Self-proclaimed as ugly, Egil possesses a distinctive appearance that seems to have been hereditary and could be classified as a form of disfigurement.

Approximately 150 years after his death, Egil's body was exhumed, and the process is described in the saga:

> They were much larger than the bones of other men. From the tales of old people it is thought pretty sure that these were Egil's bones. Skapti the priest...took then the skull of Egil, and set it on the churchyard fence. The skull was wondrous large, but still more out of the common way was its heaviness. **It was all wave-marked on the surface like a shell.** Skapti then wished to try the thickness of the skull. He took a good-sized hand-axe, and brandishing it aloft in one hand, brought down the back of it with force on the skull to break it. But where the blow fell the bone whitened, but neither was dinted nor cracked. Whence it might be gathered that this skull could not easily be harmed by the blows of weak men while skin and flesh were on it. (Ch. 89)

Byock translates the emphasized line as "ridged all over on the outside like a scallop shell," citing that the Icelandic words are "*hörpuskel* (scallop shell) and *bárótr* (ridged, waved, corrugated, wrinkled)"; he finds that these words are unusual in the Icelandic corpus, only appearing in this passage in *Egil's Saga*.[92] The other information of note in this passage is that the skull was so hard and thick that it was nearly impervious to harm, rather unusual for a skull that had been buried for over a century.

In 1984, doctor Þórður Harðarson, followed in 1993 by Byock, suggested that Egil Skallagrímsson, based on these descriptions, had Paget's disease. The National Institute of Arthritis and Musculoskeletal and Skin Diseases

90 Byock, "Egil's Bones."

91 Byock, "Skull and Bones," 25.

92 Byock, "Skull and Bones," 33.

(NIAMS) defines Paget's disease as a "chronic (long-lasting) disorder that causes bones to grow larger and become weaker than normal," which "usually affects just one or a few bones." Approximately 42% of cases affect the skull, as possibly is the case with Egil.[93] According to NIAMS, symptoms of the disease can include: increased head size and pressure on the brain, headaches and hearing loss, tingling and numbness in the arms and legs, and loosened teeth. Byock notes that scalloping or corrugation of the skull occurs in a statistically significant number of patients and that, in advanced cases, the affected bone becomes hardened, heavier, and resistant to cutting as it grows and layers abnormally.[94] These features are remarkably similar to the description of Egil's exhumed skull.

Evidence continues to build in examination of Egil in his old age. In Chapter 88 of the saga, he is described as "heavy in movement," "dull both in hearing and sight," and "stiff in the legs." It recounts instances in which Egil stumbles or finds it difficult to walk. Egil himself talks about being blind and how his feet are always cold. While, of course, many of these conditions can be explained by old age, they are also in line with those experienced with Paget's disease, especially in conjunction with age.

When we are analyzing historical evidence, it is important to remember that diagnosis can be problematic. Something like Paget's disease, while it existed, was not understood as a condition of its own in the Middle Ages. It was first described, and thus named after, English surgeon and pathologist Sir James Paget in 1877. Also, in a case like Egil, we are working from centuries-old descriptions rather than a physical body. There is always room for error. Other researchers have posited that Egil instead had skeletal fluorosis, which has similar symptoms, but also is consistent with Icelandic environmental factors.[95] Finding Egil's legendary skull might put these debates to rest, but, until then, we can only imagine.

Regardless of their cause, Egil's disfigured features seem only to enhance his reputation. In the scene in which he is described in Chapter 55, he is sitting across from King Athelstan after they have fought a battle together. Egil believes that the king owes him compensation for his brother's death. The warrior's features are made more dreadful by his anger, clearly expressing his emotions to the king who chooses to pay him rather than ignite his wrath. And certainly, his skull's remarkable resiliency was considered a

93 Ralston, "Paget's Disease of Bone," 644.

94 Byock, "Skull and Bones," 34.

95 Weinstein, "Palaeopathology by Proxy."

wonder, adding to Egil's reputation. It is not until the end of his life that Egil is gently mocked, both by others and himself, for symptoms exacerbated by age. For a warrior then, and particularly an Icelandic one, perhaps unusual features are useful.

Contexts: Ethics of Displaying the Human Body

When I was in high school, we had a field trip to a university medical research facility. The tour included a very earnest and enthusiastic graduate student leading us through the cadaver lab. I could barely listen because I was so appalled at what seemed like the casual treatment of human bodies, displayed on our behalf.

I have since realized that the ethics of fields that require interaction with human bodies are far more complex than my uneasy revulsion as a young person understood. Scientific advancement and medical discoveries require examination of human anatomy, and, although the history of this type of study is not particularly palatable, in current legitimate research, the bodies of the recently deceased are provided with the consent of the individuals. On the other hand, at the same time there are illegal and disrespectful uses of human bodies that occur in the modern day (and have certainly occurred in the past) that hover over this work.

Further, other fields of study beyond medicine also rely on human remains: for instance, archaeology. Skeletons contain a wealth of information that can allow us to understand other time periods and cultures as well as our own. However, it is important to remember that these skeletons were once humans with lives and stories of their own.

Is a Body Cultural Heritage?

First, there is the question of whether human bodies are themselves cultural heritage. The answer to this question is far from straightforward. Maria Giovanna Belcastro and Valentina Mariotti categorize human bodies into five categories: osteoarchaeological collections, scientific and medical collections, relics and religious remains, recent remains, and remains of outstanding individuals.[96] These categories may overlap depending on the circumstances. D. Gareth Jones and Robyn J. Harris assert that "skeletal remains are part of the world's heritage, since the information they yield is relevant to and may even be said to belong to all human communities."[97]

96 Belcastro and Mariotti, "The Place of Human Remains."

97 Jones and Harris, "Archaeological Human Remains," 256.

Marta Licata et al. expand on this idea: "The remains tell us how those who preceded us have lived, worked and suffered over the years and how illness (and healing) have marked their body."[98] In this argument, bodies meet the standard for cultural heritage because of their ability to educate. Yet they are human, not strictly objects, although there is an avenue of study of how bodies essentially become objects when they are collected by a museum, as they move "along the same acquisition routes as plants, animals, and books, in the process shifting from subject to object."[99] Belcastro and Mariotti note that because human remains are of archaeological interest, they are cultural heritage; however, legislations and regulations, such as those provided by UNESCO, are not explicit in defining them as such.[100] We might argue that because historical human remains are exhibited in museums, they qualify as cultural heritage; however, more and more there are concerns about the ethics of such exhibits, as demonstrated by their removal from display or their repatriation.[101]

It seems there is a general understanding that human bodies are a form of cultural heritage capable of generating a wealth of information, but how that translates to human and legal rights is ambiguous.

The Questions

There are many questions about the ethics of displaying human remains, not to mention their interpretation.[102] Licata et al. summarize:

> The requests for repatriation/restitution of funerary artifacts and human remains advanced by heirs or local communities, in the name of a unique bond or a specific identity, have progressively highlighted the breadth and complexity of the moral questions that revolve around human remains: ownership, burial, conservation and treatment, public exposure, respect for cultures, communication with the community, identification of parameters and ethical and legal references; the protection and accessibility of cultural heritage.[103]

We need to look more closely at a few of these issues.

---

98 Licata et al., "Study, Conservation and Exhibition of Human Remains."

99 Alberti, "Objects and the Museum," 563.

100 Belcastro and Mariotti, "The Place of Human Remains."

101 See Scovazzi, "Human Remains as Cultural Heritage."

102 See the JSTOR Reading List on "Human Remains and Museums": https://daily.jstor.org/human-remains-and-museums-a-reading-list/.

103 Licata et al., "Study, Conservation and Exhibition of Human Remains."

Who owns a body? Alive, a human being should have control over their own bodies, although certainly there are violations of that right on a regular basis. Once deceased, however, a body's rights become more debatable, particularly if the individual does not express their desires for the treatment of their body. If a person's immediate family is legally the owner of a body, what happens if there is no family? And especially if that body is hundreds, if not thousands, of years old, and thus an immediate family no longer exists? In some cases, descendants in the form of a person's community—if not related by genetics, then at least connected to the deceased—might have a claim. Occasionally, the museum or other institution that has custody of a particular body will know where it came from, and ownership can be identified. But what about situations in which there is no known provenance?

These questions become more important in cases where the individual is part of a minoritized or marginalized group. Stephen C. Kenny discusses the development of medical museums in the antebellum American South, particularly in how they acquired bodies and whose bodies they acquired, especially the racist use of "slaves as anatomical resources."[104] These museums "nearly always ignored the consultation of slave patients, or their families, in the process of organ removal and retention of loved ones' bodies as anatomical objects."[105] Wendi A. Lindquist details the stealing of the skull of Pacific Northwest Chinook leader Chief Comcomly and how it ended up in the collection of the museum of the Royal Naval Hospital in Haslar, England.[106] Despite knowing how the Chinook felt about disrespecting the dead, the physician at Fort Vancouver Meredith Gairdner chose to take the skull and "tried to justify the theft in the name of science, suggesting that studies of Comcomly's skull could offer valuable insights about the Chinook leader and perhaps even humans in general."[107] The Chief's skull was returned to the Chinook community in 1972 and was reinterred. These are merely two examples among countless others of particularly indigenous and Black bodies and remains that were obtained illegally and certainly without any consent of those connected to them, and Gairdner's justification for stealing Chief Comcomly's skull is uncomfortably close to the claim that skeletal remains are part of the world's heritage and thus belong to everyone.

---

104 Kenny, "Development of Medical Museums," 34.

105 Kenny, "Development of Medical Museums," 34

106 Lindquist, "Stealing from the Dead."

107 Lindquist, "Stealing from the Dead," 327.

Respect for other cultures also means respecting beliefs about the human body and, by extension, burial practices. For instance, "human remains belonging to Native Americans and Indigenous peoples may have a sacred meaning, and it is difficult for these people to treat them as 'ordinary things.'"[108] The Chinooks "ranked stealing from the dead as one of the worst crimes a person could commit."[109] These burial practices themselves are a form of cultural heritage and should be honoured.

However, sometimes, even with the best of intentions, navigating cultural beliefs can be complicated. Belcastro and Mariotti discuss the case of skeletons excavated from a medieval Jewish cemetery in Bologna, Italy. The researchers had worked with the local Jewish community, who recognized the benefits of understanding more about these people, to begin their excavations, however the more strictly orthodox Hatra Kadisha for the Preservation of Holy sites and the European Committee for the Protection of Jewish Cemeteries protested. Eventually, the bodies were reburied in a modern Jewish cemetery in Bologna before completion of the study, putting the local Jewish community at odds with these organizations and negating at least some of the benefits that could have come from it.[110]

Implications for Disabled Bodies

The disabled community is and has been a marginalized community. Like Black and indigenous peoples, they have not always been given the choice about whether their bodies will be studied or displayed. Janet E. Lord and Christopher J. Hart detail the fate of many: "Following death, disabled bodies have been victimized, whether as a consequence of undignified burials, despoilment, mutilation and public display of remains, or disappearances about which we know very little."[111] Even when consent is given by an individual, actual choice might be an illusion. Sandell et al., citing the 1797 book *Memoirs of Remarkable Persons* by J. Cauldfield, tell the story of Owen Farrel, a little person who worked as a strong man, who "sold his body to a Mr. Omrod, a surgeon, for a weekly allowance who, after his death, made a skeleton of his bones which...at present is preserved (in the museum) of the late Dr William Hunter at the University of Glasgow."[112] We can suppose that

108 Kowalski, "Legal Status of Human Remains," 148.

109 Lindquist, "Stealing from the Dead," 325.

110 Belcastro and Mariotti, "The Place of Human Remains."

111 Lord and Hart, "Disabled Dead Bodies," 6–7.

112 Sandell et al., "In the Shadow of the Freakshow."

economic concerns might have driven Farrel to make the decision to monetize his body, and we cannot know whether he was aware that his skeleton would be donated to a museum.

Further, the contextualization of disabled bodies in museums has unfortunately tended towards the "sensational" or "unusual," "reinforc[ing] a disabled person's sense of difference, rather than of belonging."[113] Medical museums, by definition, have and display disabled bodies to represent bodily differences or anomalies. At a 2022 virtual conference hosted by The Council for British Archaeology and the Chartered Institute for Archaeologists' Early Careers Special Interest Group, Roisin Mackie presented her survey of the human remains collections and exhibitions of nine UK museums. She pointed out the differences between those that provided no social context and focused exclusively on extreme cases with those that presented the lived experiences of people with disabilities and considered the individuals connected to the artifacts.[114] Mackie found that the "erasure of disabled stories and its dehumanization whether it is intentional or not...is a persistent theme in the curation of disabled human remains."[115]

Suggestions for Ethical Approaches

First and foremost, the most ethical method for the display and study of human remains is respect. It is essential not to forget the humanity and the cultures that they represent and the dignity owed to the individuals they were. As Licata et al. suggest, "exhibition[s] must take place with methods that also respect the modesty of the subject," "[d]ignity must be the rule."[116] Evolutionary anthropologist Amanda Rossillo eloquently explains:

> As paleoanthropologists, we aim to understand humanity in all its forms. Yet, we study ancient skeletons and build careers on debating their significance while ironically forgetting about the lives that these remnants represent— ancestor or not. We should take care to remember those facets of lives lost to history—the parts of humanity that will be forever beyond the grasp of science—and acknowledge that although data and interpretations may change, each piece of the puzzle has inherent value.[117]

These are humans and deserve the recognition of their humanity.

113 Sandell et al., "In the Shadow of the Freakshow."

114 Council for British Archaeology, "Overlooked But on Display."

115 Council for British Archaeology, "Overlooked But on Display," at 9 min. 40 sec.

116 Licata et al., "Study, Conservation and Exhibition of Human Remains."

117 Rossillo, "Contemplating the Lives."

There are more concrete methods that we can consider. At the King Richard III Visitor Centre in Leicester, England, despite the fact that the museum is dedicated to the archaeological dig that found Richard and the king's body, there are no human remains on display. Instead, they display a reproduction of, in particular, Richard's spine to demonstrate its curvature. With the advancements in technology, such as 3D printing, there may be an acceptable compromise that would preserve the dignity of human bodies and still serve the goal of education. In addition, such methods might respect the wishes of communities to repatriate and rebury human remains while preserving access to scientific and historical evidence. However, these are methods that would need to be discussed with those communities and certainly should not replace accurate and respectful contextualization.

My own approach in this book is perhaps another method to consider. There are benefits of an imaginary exhibition with respect to the ethics of putting human remains on display. We can examine and explore the contexts, circumstances, and stories of these bodies without exposing them to a potentially disrespectful and dehumanizing gaze.

Chapter 2

DAILY LIFE

THE NEXT SECTION of the exhibition could be conceived a bit more like a traditional museum, with a collection of different types of mobility devices and manuscripts in cases along the walls.

Section 1: Heritage of Human Ingenuity

Humans are renowned for finding solutions to situations; thus, we are always inventing ways to manage disabilities and navigate daily life. As humans, we have a need to figure out ways to approach issues that confront us. If we do not have a limb or we cannot speak, we try to find ways to accommodate those situations. This creativity is the heritage of human ingenuity.

Røldal Stave Church Hand-Trestles

Wood; Vestland, Norway, possibly fourteenth century; University Museum of Bergen, Norway

In 2019, I developed a temporary physical disability due to sciatica that affected my back. In addition to a great deal of pain, I at times had to use a cane and, during an unavoidable trip to the airport, a wheelchair. During these experiences, I could not help but think about the accommodation needs for a lack of mobility; the stares from strangers, especially at seeing a seemingly outwardly healthy woman taking up a wheelchair; and the unwarranted shame at times of having to ask for help. In particular, temporarily using a cane and a wheelchair focused my attention on mobility devices.

The type of disability a person has dictates the type of mobility device they need. If one leg is affected but not the other, then a single crutch might be the most useful. If both legs are affected, but still have some mobility, then a pair of crutches might be more appropriate. If a person is unable to propel themselves forward, then other devices are needed, such as a cart or a wheelchair.

Mobility aids are described frequently in miracle stories to emphasize the disabilities of the people coming to a location or to a saint to be treated. Once the individuals are healed, they might leave their crutch or cane as

DOI: 10.17302/asgs32686 © Arc Humanities Press

an offering, making these sites prime locations to find them.[1] There is also documentation of these mobility aids as offerings being destroyed in the Reformation, such as at Fana Church in Norway, which claimed to have a miraculous crucifix.[2]

Canes and Crutches

Canes (or walking sticks) and crutches are relatively simple yet effective pieces of technology. The principle is: if one leg is affected in some way, then reinforce or replace it with something else to stabilize the body. There are a number of crutches that have been found in archaeological excavations.[3] We also have many images of crutches in medieval manuscripts and other works of art that depict variations in design.

The Rutland Psalter (London, British Library, Add. MS 62925) from the mid-thirteenth century depicts a person with a baby on their back holding a stick with a hand grip out in front of them (similar to the fifth from the left in Fig. 8). The distance between the person and the stick indicates that it is more of a cane than a crutch, as crutches are more effectively used closer to the body. The fifteenth-century *Liber medicinarum* (London, British Library, Sloane MS 56) by John Arderne has marginalia of a person with a pair of crutches (similar to the second from the left in Fig. 8) under both arms. The fifteenth-century German *Tübinger Hausbuch* (Universitätsbibliothek Tübingen, MD 2) has a similar figure, only this pair of crutches also has hand grips. In an image of Martin of Tours in a fifteenth-century Latin Missal (London, British Library, Egerton MS 3018), a figure in the background has both a pair of crutches and a pair of knee braces similar to one found at the Røldal Stave Church, which has holes bored into it to allow a leather strap to bind it to the leg (such as the strap in the sixth from the left in Fig. 8, which was used to attach the crutch to the body).[4] The Luttrell Psalter (London, British Library, Add. MS 42130), created in England around 1320–1340, contains an image of people going to a shrine with various mobility aids, including a pair of crutches like those in the *Liber Medicinarum*, a cane or walking stick (similar to the first item in Fig. 8), and a pair of hand-trestles (the last item in Fig. 8).

---

1 See Sveinsdóttir, "A Material Culture of Medieval Disability," 51.

2 Hagen, *Miraculous Crosses and Crucifixes*, 385–86.

3 See Kahlow, "Prothesen im Mittelalter."

4 Sveinsdóttir, "A Material Culture of Medieval Disability," 51.

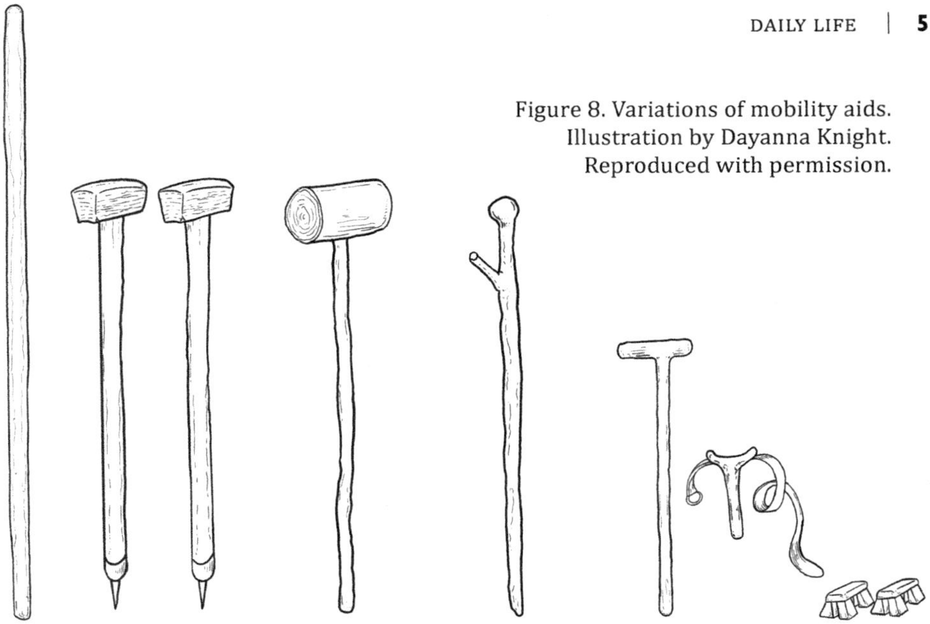

Figure 8. Variations of mobility aids. Illustration by Dayanna Knight. Reproduced with permission.

Hand-Trestles

Looking like what we would think of as mini-versions of walkers today, hand-trestles are a bit more complex in usage if not in design. Used by individuals who were compelled to move along the ground due to mobility impairments, they "provide a support and elevation for the arms, while the individual pulls themselves forwards by their upper body strength."[5] Hand-trestles served as a form of security as well as protection from the ground, and they might be used in conjunction with knee braces that could likewise insulate the joints from the terrain.

A well-known manuscript illustration is the thirteenth-century *Topographia Hiberniae* (London, British Library, Royal MS 13 B VIII) written by Gerald of Wales around 1188. The man is depicted moving along the ground, his legs at abnormal angles, propelling himself with the help of the trestles. The *Book of the Foundation of St. Bartholomew's Church*, written in Latin and translated to Middle English around 1400–1425, describes miracles that occurred at Saint Bartholomew's Church and Hospital in London. In this text, a carpenter named Wolmer is severely disabled to the point that he moves by supporting himself on "two little stools" as "he dragged behind him the heavy weight of his body."[6] It is likely these stools are hand-trestles.

5 Sveinsdóttir, "A Material Culture of Medieval Disability," 49.

6 *Book of the Foundation of St. Bartholomew's Church*, ed. King and Barnard, 12.

In the study by Anne-Marie Bouttiaux and Marc Ghysels about the Djenné terracotta figures dating from the thirteenth to the seventeenth centuries, they also identify three statues depicting "a disabled man moving about on his knees, supporting himself with semi-circular crutches in his hands."[7] As these figures share characteristics with those of the Scrofulous Sogolon, indicating a possible connection between mother and son, they have associated these with representations of the Emperor of Mali Sundiata.[8] Bouttiaux and Ghysels note that "[a]part from the kneeling position with ring crutches signaling disablement, another interesting feature is that almost all visual details in these sculptures suggest a man who will later stand up on his own. His power is immanent and the figures seem filled with determination."[9] This posture reflects the descriptions of Sundiata's disabilities and his subsequent recovery. The semi-circular ring crutches are similar in design to hand-trestles.

The hand-trestles found at Røldal Stave Church—a wooden church built in 1250 in Vestland, Norway—also known, like Fana Church, for its miracle-working crucifix, are unique in their design: "rather than the handle being supported by individual wooden poles, it has a flat under-lying surface, which would have affected the trestle's grip."[10] This flat surface may have provided more stability than the traditional design. These particular trestles, thought to date approximately to the fourteenth century, were objects of offering left at the church along with a collection of body part-shaped votives that also could represent people with disabilities coming to the church for miraculous healing: "A devotee seeking miraculous healing would in some cases provide an anatomical votive, i.e. a replica of their affected body part, to be left at a shrine."[11] The finding and study of hand-trestles is important for medieval disability heritage, "provid[ing] an insight into the embodied experience of individuals with lower limb impairment through the material affordances of these objects."[12]

---

7 Bouttiaux and Ghysels, "Scrofulous Sogolon," 101.

8 See Chapter 1 for more on Sundiata's disabilities.

9 Bouttiaux and Ghysels, "Scrofulous Sogolon," 101.

10 Sveinsdóttir, "A Material Culture of Medieval Disability," 49.

11 Sveinsdóttir, "A Material Culture of Medieval Disability," 40.

12 Sveinsdóttir, "A Material Culture of Medieval Disability," 55.

Time and Space

My experience using a cane and a wheelchair reinforced with me one particular aspect of disability: the relationship with time. Alicia Spencer-Hall defines *crip time* as the "time of disability, but also the times—plural—made possible by disability, the times in excess of the normate," as a phrase "challenging linguistic and significative stability by insisting on difference, different ways of doing, being, and thinking."[13] Amelia Kennedy contrasts crip time with *normate time*, "the socially sanctioned temporal rhythms governing presumptively able-bodied lives, rhythms that emphasize productivity and conform to 'work time,' 'clock time,' or 'institutional time.'" An example of crip time, as Dominika Bednarska outlines, is the expenditure of limited energy and the decisions concerning how to spend energy in contrast to expected levels of productivity.[14] Amelia Kennedy has looked at crip time in medieval monasteries, finding that infirmaries were spaces that "offered a pause from the normate regular time of the canonical hours and other daily duties."[15]

The way time manifests for those experiencing disability varies greatly—sometimes negatively, neutrally, or positively, and sometimes all three at once. Using mobility devices changes a person's relationship with time. For instance, although they assist in mobility or perhaps even make mobility possible at all, it takes longer to move with a pair of crutches. A person may not even be able to navigate the most direct way to a destination if that route is not accessible to a device. Perhaps the ground is more uneven or there are steps. Not to mention the pain that movement with such disabilities might entail. Thus, the time it takes to complete a task or to travel is different for someone with such a disability.

Consider also the concept of space. For those who used the hand-trestles, their view of the world was from the ground, looking up with the lower bodies of others at eye level. They themselves were not at the eye level of most people, except perhaps children, hindering their immediate visibility in any space. These circumstances would change a person's relationship with their environment.

---

13 Spencer-Hall, "Stopping the Clock(s)."

14 Bednarska, "Rethinking Access," 165.

15 Kennedy, "Crip Time in the Medieval Monasteries," 72.

"Spring on the Yellow River" with "Enlargement of Seeing-eye Dog"

Scroll; China, approximately 1250; Reproduction owned Perkins School for the Blind Samuel P. Hayes Research Library, Watertown, MA, courtesy of the Metropolitan Museum of Art

The Blind in Art Collection of the Perkins School for the Blind's Samuel P. Hayes Research Library brings together images—largely reproductions—of the "history of blindness, stereotypes, and depictions from other aspects of popular culture and the media."[16] In this collection, there is a reproduction of a thirteenth-century Chinese scroll.[17] The original is in the Metropolitan Museum of Art. What is interesting about the Perkins copy is that it also includes an "Enlargement of Seeing-eye Dog" next to the main image with a caption. In this inset, the focus is on a person hunched over, carrying a cane in their right hand, with the stick pointing out in front of them, and a leash attached to a dog being held in the other. Given the position of the cane and the seeming infirmity of the individual, this person is understood to be visually impaired, and the logical conclusion is that the dog is assisting them to navigate.

While the first official guide dog training school did not open until 1916 in Germany—with the first in the United States, the Seeing Eye, opening in 1929—there has been a long tradition of the Blind and assistance dogs, with one of the oldest images appearing in a wall painting at Pompeii.[18]

Medieval Guide Dogs[19]

The evidence for medieval guide dogs is extensive. Krista A. Milne has compiled a collection of manuscript illustrations with individuals being led by dogs. An illustration from the French manuscript of the Smithfield Decretals, or the Decretals of Gregory IX, from the thirteenth century (London, British Library, Royal MS 10 E IV) has a person with clear patches in their clothing wearing a hat and a bag slung around their body. They are leaning on the walking stick in their left hand (similar to the first item in Fig. 8) and holding on to a leash in their right hand. This leash is tied to a brown dog in front of

16 See Perkins School for the Blind, "Blind in Art Collection."

17 Perkins School for the Blind, "Spring on the Yellow River."

18 See Ostermeier, "History of Guide Dog use."

19 This section draws mainly from Krista A. Milne's work, especially her blog post "Guide Dogs in Medieval Art and Writing," which was a precursor to her *Textual and Artistic Representations of Guide Dogs in Northwestern Europe, 1100 to 1500*, forthcoming from Palgrave.

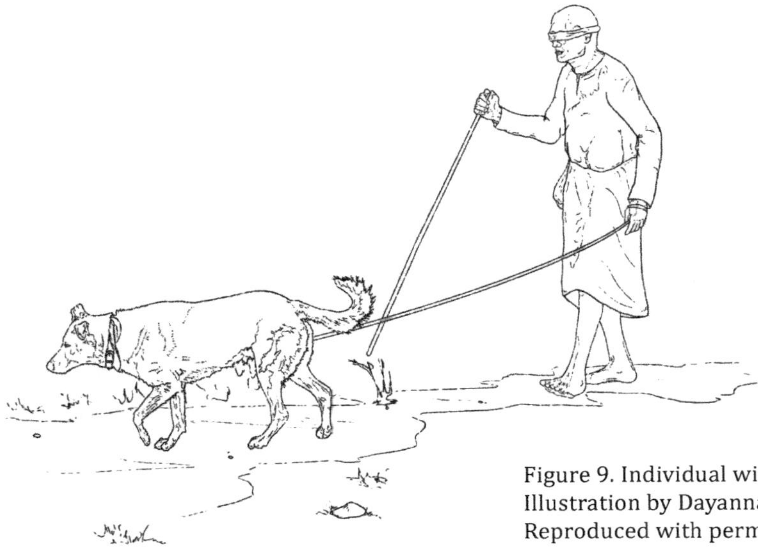

Figure 9. Individual with guide dog. Illustration by Dayanna Knight. Reproduced with permission.

the person; the dog's nose is high in the air, appearing to almost pull on its tether tied around its neck. The dog is particularly sturdy and seems rather intent on its mission. The individual's eyes are closed, and they have a far less sure expression than their canine companion. Figure 9 shows an artistic rendering of a similar scene.

A fourteenth-century Book of Hours (London, British Library, Stowe MS 17) contains a scene in which Christ is healing a Blind person, who stands with their hands clasped in prayer. Stretching from them is a leash that connects behind to the neck of a white dog, who is sitting and watching the proceedings with seeming excitement or anticipation.

Another Book of Hours (Baltimore, Walters Art Museum, MS 82) produced in Ghent, also in the fourteenth century, has a very active illustration of another person with a walking stick like that in the Smithfield Decretals; their eyes are looking upwards, away from the action in front of them, indicating blindness. They are being pulled forward by a white dog on a leash as the animal runs up the side of the illustration, carrying a bowl in its mouth. Milne notes that there are other examples of guide dogs with bowls that perhaps are representative of the dogs seeking alms for their humans.

In terms of textual evidence of guide dogs, Milne points to a passage by Nikephoros Basilakes, a rhetoric teacher in twelfth-century Constantinople. In his "Encomium" about dogs, he says, "Why do I not mention the most unusual characteristic of all, that he leads the blind and becomes another eye for them, and that he leads them around everywhere to beg for bread at people's doors, and then leads them back again to their lodging?"[20] We do have

20 Nikephoros Basilakes, "Encomium," 136–37.

other texts that claim dogs are too easily distracted to make good guides, but perhaps these are by individuals with less experience with the animals.

Training and Roles of Dogs

Animals were a ubiquitous part of life in the Middle Ages. They were modes of transportation, they provided and helped to grow sustenance, and they provided entertainment. Dogs were a particularly prevalent animal in medieval Europe. For the nobility, they served as hunting companions. Written in England between 1406 and 1413 by Edward III's grandson Edward, the second Duke of York, *The Master of the Game* is a treatise on hunting. Edward writes:

> A hound is true to his lord and his master, and of good love and true. A hound is of great understanding and of great knowledge, a hound hath great strength and great goodness, a hound is a wise beast and a kind (one). A hound has a great memory and great smelling, a hound has great diligence and great might, a hound is of great worthiness and of great subtlety, a hound is of great lightness and of great perseverance (?), a hound is of good obedience, for he will learn as a man all that a man will teach him.[21]

In this passage, the author emphasizes that dogs can be wise creatures and are able to be taught, which are useful characteristics for guide dogs, as are loyalty and diligence. We see this respect for a dog-like creature's actions in Marie de France's late twelfth-century lai *Bisclavret*, in which the title character turns into a wolf but is taken in and honoured by the king for his impeccable behaviour.[22]

In his *De animalibus*, the thirteenth-century Dominican friar and philosopher Albertus Magnus discusses dogs, particularly for hunting, guarding, and entertaining. He details fairly extensively the training required for each of these roles, the guidance at times seemingly close to modern ideas for training. He comments that dogs can be taught almost anything, although certain ones are more suited in personality for such work as hunting and guarding.[23] Archaeological studies of dogs from Estonia indicate that there were working dogs, stray dogs—which served to help clean up waste in urban environments—and pets or companions.[24]

---

21 Edward of Norwich, *The Master of Game*, ed. Baillie-Grohman and Baillie-Grohman, ch. 12. Project Gutenberg, 2024. https://www.gutenberg.org/files/43452/43452-h/43452-h.htm.

22 See Crane, *Animal Encounters.*

23 Krause, Ganslosser, and Hohlfeld, "Dog Training, Keeping and Selection."

24 Nuut et al., "Pets or Functional Animals."

The use of dogs in the military and war is difficult to trace. According to Gervase Phillips, in the medieval period they were more likely "dogs in war" rather than "dogs of war," fulfilling similar functions to guarding. By the late Middle Ages, there is clearer documentation:

> By the later fifteenth century...the proliferation of both printed literature and administrative documentation gives us yet greater, and more reliable, evidence. This includes some suggestions of long-standing, but probably localised, traditions of employing dogs in military and quasi-military contexts, especially in the familiar roles of sentry.[25]

It does not seem that they were trained in any systematic way to participate in military actions.

Animals were considered pets or, as Kathleen Walker-Meikle defines them, "animals chosen by humans simply to perform the task of being companions."[26] The Prioress in Geoffrey Chaucer's fourteenth-century *Canterbury Tales* has some small hounds that she feeds on roasted flesh, milk, and bread (*General Prologue*, lines 146–47),[27] their size indicating they are not hunting dogs, but companions. The smallest skeleton of a dog found in Viljand, Estonia, might have been a companion dog.[28]

The presence of guide dogs in the Middle Ages indicates both the necessity to find ways for Blind people to navigate as well as the long history of relationships between animals and humans. That they are frequently included in manuscript illustrations and artworks, at least in Europe and Asia, provides evidence that they had a common place in everyday life.

STORIES: Communicating with Monastic Sign Language

Many in modern American culture assume that there is one sign language, one system of signs. On the contrary, however, American Sign Language (ASL) is only one of many. In fact, there are presently over three hundred sign languages around the world, some used in wider contexts and some that are localized to confined areas. For instance, there are "village sign languages" that develop in areas with high percentages of congenital deafness, such as Martha's Vineyard Sign Language (MVSL) used from the early eighteenth century to 1952. These are, unlike national sign languages, "typically

25 Phillips, "The Employment of War Dogs," 6.

26 Walker-Meikle, *Medieval Pets*, ix.

27 All references to *The Canterbury Tales* taken from: Geoffrey Chaucer, *The Canterbury Tales and Other Works*, http://www.librarius.com/.

28 Nuut et al., "Pets or Functional Animals," 98.

shared between deaf and hearing community members, thus facilitating a high degree of integration between deaf and hearing individuals."[29] There are also types of communication by sign that can range from gestural or rudimentary to a systematic language. Many speakers tend to gesture when they talk, but "gesture systems do not possess self-standing grammar"; however, "non-linguistic gestural systems [can and do] become linguistic over time."[30] A simple method used by an individual or family to communicate can develop into a sophisticated language system.

Language in general is a part of cultural heritage. As Bruno de Witte writes, "The use of a particular language not only serves as a means of functional communication but also expresses the speaker's cultural identity, as well as the cultural heritage developed by all previous users of that language."[31] Many users of sign language are keenly aware of their language's significance. Jody Barney—an Aboriginal woman from Queensland, Australia—was born deaf and knows eighteen indigenous sign languages. She comments on that pride: "Aboriginal sign language systems, they're expressive, they're visual, they're culturally bound, they're old. Their value is priceless… the signs that I use today are the same signs that have been used for 65,000 years."[32] While sign languages are used by and to communicate with Deaf people and communities, there are other reasons they might develop, such as cultural taboos or necessity.

One such necessity existed in monastic communities in the Middle Ages, especially in the cenobitic communities that practised vows of silence, which presented a need for some form of communication. Rather than only gestural, these signs developed into formal systems of language, among them Old English, Augustinian, Benedictine, and Cistercian. We are not certain as to exact dates when sign language was first used by monastic orders, but "there is every indication that most of the early orders specified the use of signs when and where verbal communication was not desirable."[33] Likely, this preference for signs came about because, as Scott G. Bruce states, "silence emerged as an important aspect of monastic conduct in the earliest days of Christian asceticism, the first principle of which was the renunciation of the world in anticipation of the Last Judgment"; thus "early medieval

29 de Vos and Zeshan, "Introduction," 2.

30 Brentari, *Sign Languages,* 3.

31 de Witte, "Language as Cultural Heritage," 371.

32 Murphy, "Aboriginal Sign Languages."

33 Barakat, "Cistercian Sign Language," 88.

monks were instructed to renounce any spoken words that mired their thoughts in the world and distracted their attention from God."[34] According to sources from Cluny, an influential monastery in France founded in 910 and known for its strict codes of behaviour, "conversation was prohibited in the church, the dormitory, the refectory and the kitchens," all communal areas, and "talking at night was also strictly forbidden."[35] Sign language thus became an avenue of practical communication, particularly when a person needed food.

In his study of the sign language used at Cluny, Bruce differentiates the system developed there as more than gestural:

> In the early tenth century, the strict speech prohibitions of the Cluniacs required monks to express ever more complex concerns without talking and consequently shaped a more detailed and accurate system of manual communication. Unlike the nonverbal cues employed in other abbeys, the signs described in the Life of Odo were exacting instruments of language. John of Salerno referred to them specifically as *notae*, meaning "marks" or "characters." This term was a more precise qualification than the ambiguous *signum*, because it implied that each sign carried a specific value or meaning. In contrast to arbitrary signals, the Cluniac sign language was a manual code of symbolic characters that allowed the brethren to articulate their needs with the same precision as the tongue.[36]

In general, these signs were inspired or influenced by a visual component of what they signified. Diane Brentari uses the concept of *iconicity* in language, when the word or sign mimics what it is referencing, to explain this aspect of sign language and remarks that "even though iconicity never disappears from sign languages, it is generally weakened over time."[37] Novices were formally instructed in monastic sign language, including warnings not to engage in "idle" signing that would defeat the purpose of the rule of silence. Robert A. Barakat describes how the Cistercian Sign Language is still used in modern houses, albeit influenced by local spoken vernaculars, with the official Cistercian Order's sign list deriving from a fifteenth-century one.[38]

Monastic sign language provides an interesting example of accessibility. While the main purpose of its development was spiritual protection, the

34 Bruce, *Silence and Sign Language*, 13.

35 Bruce, *Silence and Sign Language*, 26.

36 Bruce, *Silence and Sign Language*, 62.

37 Brentari, *Sign Languages*, 12.

38 Barakat, "On Ambiguity," 276–77.

common use of sign language was, no doubt, highly beneficial for monks with hearing loss, particularly as a result of aging. The same is true for those who were unable to speak for any reason, either permanently or temporarily. These disabilities would have been unremarkable and would not have been a social barrier in an environment in which silence and sign language were normalized.

Section 2: Communities of Disability

Edward Wheatley, in his *Stumbling Blocks Before the Blind: Medieval Constructions of a Disability*, describes the creation of a community for the blind in thirteenth-century France:

> In 1256, a watershed moment occurred in the history of blindness in Europe: Louis IX, better known today as Saint Louis, founded a residential hospice for the blind called the Hospice des Quinze-Vingts (literally, the Hospice of Fifteen Twenties, signifying the 300 residents whom it was meant to house). Associated with the National Center for Ophthalmology in Paris, this institution still survives today. For the residents the hospice offered basic care and some protection on the streets of Paris... It was not a hospital in which clerics took care of residents, but rather a community in which the blind and their sighted relatives lived and worked together on every aspect of communal life, from agriculture to governance.[39]

Wheatley refers to two different types of communities of disability. One is what we could classify as institutional, in which individuals are more patients or even inmates, receiving care, sometimes with consent and sometimes against their will. The second includes areas in which those with disabilities or with a specific disability gather in a more autonomous environment. The Hospice des Quinze-Vingts, for instance, "exemplified some problematic aspects of institutionalized care," but "it offered its residents relative freedom in comparison to many institutions, both medieval and modern."[40] Both types had their own purposes and their own place in medieval disability heritage.

---

39 Wheatley, *Stumbling Blocks Before the Blind*, 42–43.

40 Wheatley, *Stumbling Blocks Before the Blind*, x.

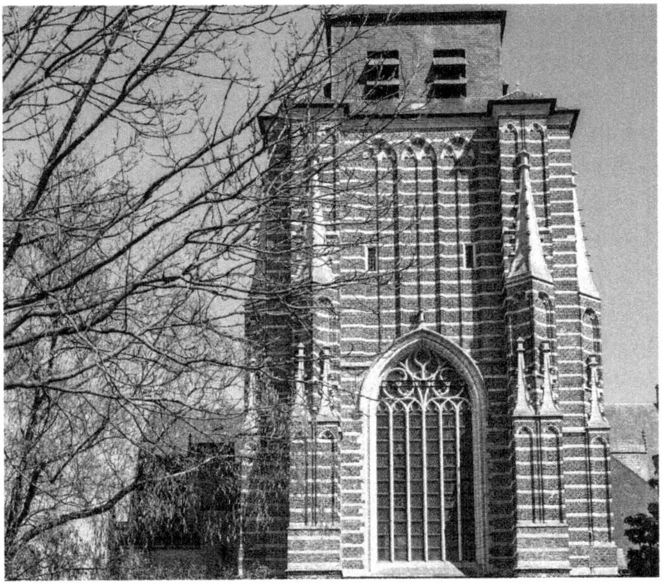

Figure 10. Sint-Dimpnakerk, Geel, Belgium. Photograph by author.

Mental Health Community in Geel

Shared Living Community; Belgium, fourteenth century to the present

The medieval saint Dymphna (Dimphna) is a legendary, seventh-century Irish princess who avoided an incestuous marriage to her father by running away to Geel, Belgium, only to be found and martyred. She became the patron saint of mental health, and her life and story became the cornerstone for the development of a mental health community of practice in Geel in the fourteenth and fifteenth centuries (see Fig. 10). Individuals, inspired by stories of mental health aid—divine and otherwise—arrived in the city to receive spiritual and physical care. This care developed into a community shared living program, one that continues today and has informed similar practices around the world. This influence has occurred despite certain criticisms by members of the medical community, particularly due to the rise of medicalization and psychiatry as an accepted medical field as well as with the dominance of the medical model of disability. The Geel community-based care model was added to the UNESCO Register of Good Safeguarding Practices in 2023 for promoting the "complementarity of diverse health care approaches by nurturing a warm-hearted ecosystem where cultural and health care practices and medical institutions merge."[41]

---

41 "Safeguarding foster care heritage in the merciful city of Geel."

Saint Dymphna's Story

Saint Dymphna's personal story is a tragic one. Her pagan Irish father, distraught at his wife's death, turned amorous attentions on his daughter and began pressuring her to marry him. Understandably, Dymphna was not receptive to this incestuous relationship, and she managed to flee to Belgium with her confessor, Gerebernus. Eventually, they landed in Geel and settled in for a simple life. Unfortunately, Dymphna's father was relentless in his pursuit and eventually found her. When Gerebernus tried to intervene, the king had him killed. At Dymphna's continued resistance to marrying him, in a fit of anger, the father beheaded his daughter himself.[42]

As stories of miracles at the site of Dymphna's death began to circulate and more people visited, she was beatified and then canonized in 1247. In the mid- to late thirteenth century was the first written account of her *Life*, authored by Belgian canon Peter van Kamerijk (Peter of Cambrai), with other versions coming later. The version in London, British Library, Stowe MS 949 recounts how "possessed persons brought to her shrine at Ghele are daylie deliuered," revealing how in particular those with mental health conditions were miraculously healed.[43] Saints are often believed to be particularly adept at certain requests, such as the curing of a specific disease or intercession for specific actions. Quite often, these were attributed to linguistic or iconographic associations.[44] In the case of Dymphna, her connection to mental health appears to be more related to her father's behaviour and an oft-circulated addendum to the story that her father was miraculously "cured" of his madness after killing his daughter.

The Geel Model of Care

As the Dymphna story grew, so did the system of care provided in Geel. Her *Life* records that "when this village was greatly peopled, and for many dwellers very famous, by reason of the wonderful cures they made happen."[45] People began arriving in such numbers that eventually, in 1349, a new church was built to accommodate them. In 1480, an additional sick room was added, and, from there, further buildings were constructed.

---

42 Taken from Horstmann's edition of London, British Library, Stowe MS 949 (ca. 1610–1615), *The Lives of Women Saints*.

43 Horstmann, *The Lives of Women Saints*, 49.

44 See Buterin, Muzur, and Glažar, "Saints and 'Possession.'"

45 Horstmann, *The Lives of Women Saints*, 47. Translations mine.

Treatment for these pilgrims was holistic—that is, they were viewed as whole human beings, rather than exclusively spiritual or medical ones, reflecting the "bodymind" philosophy that the mind and body are intrinsically interconnected. Given Dymphna's influence, there was a spiritual element to their treatment, which included being in the presence of the saint's reliquary. Dymphna's relics were discovered in the fourteenth century and include two stone sarcophagi, three thigh bones, and a jawbone. Later radiocarbon analysis dates the thigh bones and the sarcophagi fragments to the seventh or eighth century and the jaw bone to the tenth century. Discovered near the believed location of Dymphna's death, local legend dubbed them as hers and her confessor's.[46] These relics became central to the spiritual treatment of pilgrims. The physical treatment took place in the sick room and hospital. Social treatment came in the form of integration into the local community.

The number of pilgrims arriving in Geel were often greater than even the growing number of community buildings could manage. Thus, the medieval people of Geel began boarding these guests in their homes, feeding and housing them as they received treatment. These boarders would frequently stay for a long period of time and, some, for their whole lives. They would do what they were capable of doing, working, helping, socializing as they were able. They became integrated into the fabric of the village, living and mingling with the residents. These shared living practices were so effective that they have continued to today and have influenced other global methods of care, encouraging an integrative model of care that meets individuals where they are. As Hench P. J. G. Van Bilsen remarks:

> There are expectations, but no demands. Patients are allowed to function on their optimal level. If someone is capable of "pottering around" in the garden of the foster family then that is OK; just as it is OK for another patient to join the local football club. Accepting what is, not demanding what should be, seems to be the motto.[47]

Indeed, "praised by the World Health Organization, the town of Geel (Belgium) and its family care tradition, rooted in the [M]iddle [A]ges and largely avoiding the blight of institutionalization, is an exemplary model of social inclusion."[48]

---

46 See Haneca and Buyle, "The Reliquary of Saint Dymphna."

47 Van Bilsen, "Lessons to Be Learned," 209.

48 McCrary, "Geel's Family Care Tradition," 285–86.

A Parallel in Iwakura, Japan

A parallel story to Geel exists in eleventh-century Iwakura near Kyoto, Japan. Like its Belgian counterpart, Iwakura's story begins in legend. Experiencing a mental health issue, the daughter of Emperor Go-Sanjō, who ruled from 1034 to 1073, travelled to the Daiunji Temple in Iwakura. After praying to the image of Kannon, the Buddhist deity of mercy, and drinking the water from the temple well, she was miraculously cured. Others began following her example, coming to the temple for mental health treatment.[49] Kannon appears in other Japanese stories of disability, such as the story of "A Woman Who Could Not Speak Is Healed, Owing to the Grace of the Kannon of Ishiyama" in the *Konjaku Monogatari Shu*, written approximately 794 to 1185.

It is unlikely that the legend of the emperor's daughter is factual, but rather was promoted by Daiunji in the middle of the eighteenth century to encourage travel to the temple. By the end of that century, Iwakura had certainly "established its reputation for healing mentally ill patients."[50] After that time, like Geel, the number of individuals seeking treatment increased dramatically, stretching their resources thin, and, inspired by the Belgian city, Dr. Eikichi Tsuchiya, the director of Iwakura Mental Hospital, "not only promoted 'Iwakura' as 'a Geel in Japan,' but urged the neighbors around the hospital to establish residential sanatoria."[51] Unfortunately, the family care system in Iwakura closed during World War II, due to shortages of food and re-purposing by the Japanese army.

Geel's Legacy

Centuries of community integration have created a space in Geel in which experiencing mental health issues is normalized. While Geel neither was nor is a utopia, its existence is evidence that those with mental health issues in the Middle Ages were not always treated negatively and that we can learn from premodern approaches to holistic care.

---

49 See Hashimoto, "The Invention of a 'Japanese Gheel.'"

50 Nakamura, "Family Care of Mentally Ill Patients," 98.

51 Nakamura, "Family Care of Mentally Ill Patients," 99.

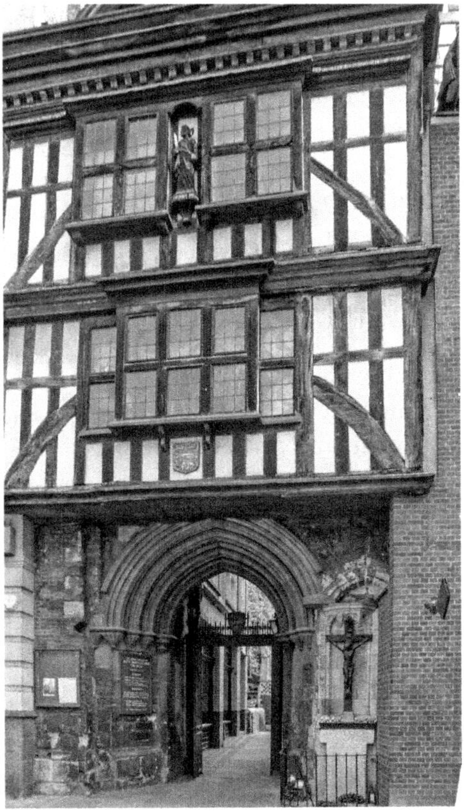

Figure 11. Original nave of Saint Bartholomew the Great, London. Photograph by author.

Saint Bartholomew's Church and Hospital

West Smithfield, London, founded 1123

Founded in 1123, Saint Bartholomew the Great's Church and Hospital is London's oldest surviving parish church (see Fig. 11). It is an example of a medieval hospital, of which there were many in medieval England and Wales. Typically, they were allied with an accompanying religious centre and generally treated patients of all kinds, including those with disabilities. While medical and spiritual treatments were prescribed in these hospitals, in some ways they served more as communities of care for those in need, either temporarily or for longer periods of time. Saint Bartholomew's served as "almshouses for the elderly and infirm" and "places for pilgrims to rest," in addition to "taking in orphans and children of unmarried mothers and providing them with care and schooling" as well as general "medical care."[52]

The Founding Story

The founding story of the church and hospital is recorded in the *Book of the Foundation of St. Bartholomew's Church.*[53] Like the story of Geel, a saint is heavily involved in its legendary foundation. After living a life of worldly endeavors as a courtier, a man named Rahere decided to change his ways and journey to Rome. While on this journey, he became very ill, and, in fear of his life, he promised God that he would found a hospital if he recovered—a request that was granted. One night after his recovery, Rahere had a strange dream that ended with a conversation with Saint Bartholomew,

52 Barts Health Archives, "Research Guide."

53 The following summary and subsequent references to miracles are made from the modern translation of the *Book of the Foundation of St. Bartholomew's Church*, ed. King and Barnard.

one of Christ's Apostles. Bartholomew told Rahere that he had picked out a location in Smithfield, London, for a church. He would provide the funds and patronage, and Rahere would administer it.

Upon returning to London, Rahere consulted his many friends, including King Henry I, from whom he received permission to proceed with both the church and the hospital. Although previously prophesied to be holy ground by King Edward the Confessor, the land that Saint Bartholomew had chosen was swampy and downtrodden, fit only for the hanging of thieves. Rahere expended great effort in cleaning it up, both his own labour and that of others he organized to help. After experiencing animosity and jealousy, Rahere returned to the king and received royal patronage and protection for the church.

The Disability Miracles of Saint Bartholomew

Saint Bartholomew, as one of the Apostles, was considerably revered. Relics associated with him appeared in various locations, including eventually in Rome and San Bartolomeo all'Isola, which stands on the site of the ancient temple to Aesculapius, the Greek god of medicine, creating a link between Bartholomew and hospitals. The *Book of the Foundation* describes in detail the miracles that occurred at Saint Bartholomew's church and hospital, both during the life of Rahere and afterwards. These miracles range from the curing of animals and the finding of a stolen manuscript to the healing of various diseases.

There are a number of disabilities described in the *Book*, some rather extreme. A man named Adwyn was

> so crippled that he had not the free use either of feet or hands. Indeed, with his calves cleaving to his thighs he could not walk at all, and with his hands bent backward he could do no work; he could scarcely carry food to his mouth with just the tip of his fingers, which, too, the stiffness of his sinews had crippled.[54]

Another, Osbern, had his "right hand clave to his left shoulder, but his head lay immovable, pressed down upon his hand, and neither his hand from his shoulder, nor his head from his hand could be severed."[55] Wolmer was "oppressed with a grievous and long-standing disease, appeared wretched and pitiable to all that beheld him, for his feet hung destitute of natural vigour, his legs clave to his thighs, part of his fingers was twisted back to his

54 *Book of the Foundation of St. Bartholomew's Church*, ed. King and Barnard, 18.

55 *Book of the Foundation of St. Bartholomew's Church*, ed. King and Barnard, 15.

hand." He is described as supporting himself on "two little stools," perhaps hand trestles, as "he dragged behind him the heavy weight of his body."[56] Another girl was "deaf and dumb and deprived of the light of both eyes, and crippled with legs bent backward."[57] There are others who are mute and blind from birth, others with dropsy, epilepsy, and paralysis.

Mental disability is common in these stories as well, although more in the second book, which focuses on the miracles after the death of Rahere. A young man by the name of Robert, having encountered some sort of supernatural being while asleep, "lost his wits and was deprived of the power of reason, and, knowing not what ought to be done and what left undone, under the influence of madness he ran wandering about, now this way and now that, and, not knowing what he was doing."[58] A knight "leapt raving from the horse whereon he had sat and rent his garments in pieces, scattered the coins he was carrying, and began to assault with stones those whom he met."[59] The beautiful illegitimate daughter of Wymond the priest has a rather complicated story, in which she daily resists the devil eventually to be "afflicted in mind," "tortured with dreadful suffering of body and, rolling backwards and forwards with inordinate movements of her limbs," and "foaming at the mouth."[60] Collectively, these stories detail some of the behaviours associated with extreme mental disability.

One story is particularly noteworthy. It details how a young woman is persuaded to become a prostitute and, as a result of this sin, experiences mental illness:

> And soon the wages of sin followed, and she who prostituted her flesh lost utterly her soundness of mind, and the limbs which were the weapons of sin were turned into weapons of madness [here and in other parts of the passage, "woodness" in the Middle English]...in her punishment she comprehended neither God nor herself. Her eyes were at one time strained upwards; at another they rolled terribly; her clothes were rent by her hands; her tongue was unbridled in blasphemy, shamelessness, and inanity. As her madness increased, she was confined in stricter bonds, and when those were easily burst by her fury others were added, and thus she was carried

---

56 *Book of the Foundation of St. Bartholomew's Church*, ed. King and Barnard, 12. See Chapter 2's section "Section 1: Heritage of Human Ingenuity" for more on hand-trestles.

57 *Book of the Foundation of St. Bartholomew's Church*, ed. King and Barnard, 22.

58 *Book of the Foundation of St. Bartholomew's Church*, ed. King and Barnard, 28.

59 *Book of the Foundation of St. Bartholomew's Church*, ed. King and Barnard, 29.

60 *Book of the Foundation of St. Bartholomew's Church*, ed. King and Barnard, 31.

> to the hospital of the aforesaid church. A contraction of her limbs followed shortly after, so that she could nowise use them freely.[61]

The woman's disability is clearly allied with sin here, as participation in prostitution is the direct cause. Fury and anger are emphasized as well, even to the point where she breaks the bonds that are used to restrain her. Restraint and force are depicted frequently in these stories: the young man discussed previously was "captured," and the knight was "taken, though resisting much." She exhibits many of the characteristics in the other stories: tearing her clothes, incomprehensible speech, etc. Also, this mental distress leads to physical disability with the "contraction of her limbs."

No matter the disability or the circumstances, in all cases, regardless of the culpability of the person, these individuals are healed. The Apostle intercedes on their behalf once they are physically in the space of Saint Bartholomew's.

Church vs. Hospital

The *Book of the Foundation* seems to make a careful distinction between when the individuals needing care are brought to the church and when they are brought to the hospital. As Nicole Rice notes, the *Book of the Foundation* "tends to privilege the priory church as the site of Saint Bartholomew's miracles, but in this story [of the prostitute] the hospital is specifically mentioned as the site of his intervention."[62] When the young woman is brought to Saint Bartholomew's, "she was carried to the hospital of the aforesaid church." Adwyn as well is brought to the hospital: "Because he was far from the said church, he paid the passage money and was set on a ship and, being carried to the church, was set in the hospital of the poor and supported there some time of the alms of the said church."[63] The difference appears to be when individuals require more time for their care. Those healed immediately by prayer are taken to the church, but those who need more convalesce to the hospital. After arriving at Saint Bartholomew's, Adwyn "began to revive and his longed-for health began to return bit by bit."[64] In the case of the woman, she is described as developing the "contraction of her limbs" after she is taken to Saint Bartholomew's, implying she was there for a period of time.

---

61 *Book of the Foundation of St. Bartholomew's Church*, ed. King and Barnard, 36.

62 Rice, *The Medieval Hospital*, 53.

63 *Book of the Foundation of St. Bartholomew's Church*, ed. King and Barnard, 18.

64 *Book of the Foundation of St. Bartholomew's Church*, ed. King and Barnard, 18.

The Community at Saint Bartholomew's

The miracle stories give us a sense of the community that existed in the church and the hospital. At the beginning of its foundation, Rahere must gather people to help him build it. In the story of Godric the butcher, Rahere brings in an older man by the name of Alfune, who had experience with the administration of churches. His jobs are "to seek necessaries for the relief of the poor who lay in the hospital and of those who were hired for building the church...and faithfully to bring home what was entrusted to him and to divide it amongst them as each had need."[65] This passage demonstrates the work needed to manage the operations of Saint Bartholomew's: the people building it, the patrons who fund its operations, the merchants of the town who contribute food and other goods, in addition to the people who were seeking assistance. Further, other individuals are mentioned in the stories, particularly families. The multi-disabled girl was accompanied by her "weeping parents" who "lay clinging to the pavement and ceased not from prayer." Another little boy who "had lost all sense of reason" is brought by his mother and described as "burdensome" to her and "past bearing with." These examples emphasize the physical and emotional toll of being a caregiver, but also how disability is communal.

Stories: Living in the Mont-aux-Malades Leprosarium

Rouen, France, Twelfth Century

Known as Hansen's disease today, leprosy—a bacterial infection—is characterized by "large skin sores, and, ultimately, degeneration of the facial features, particularly the nose and palate, and destruction of the nerves at the bodily extremities, such as the fingers and toes, resulting in loss of sensation and thus damage to these areas."[66] Treatments included "modification of diet, bathing in hot springs, the use of drugs, bloodletting, avoidance of sexual activity and segregation in leprosaria [or communities dedicated to this disease]."[67] It is a disease generally associated with the Middle Ages, often making an appearance in medieval films and other medieval-esque media. These representations usually depict negative treatment of lepers, but the truth is far more complex.

---

65 *Book of the Foundation of St. Bartholomew's Church*, ed. King and Barnard, 16.

66 Brenner, *Leprosy and Charity*, 3.

67 Hamilton, *The Leper King and His Heirs*, 254.

The Representation of Lepers

As Elsa Brenner writes,

> the leprous had a special religious status in the Middle Ages, being believed to have been chosen by God to be redeemed, and were thus the objects of sympathy and compassion.... Nonetheless, it is clear that in some instances lepers were overtly marginalised, and that concern about leprosy and contagion was a factor as early as the thirteenth century, becoming more widespread in the fourteenth.[68]

She notes the connection between lepers and charity, and that giving to individuals or to leper colonies was a sure way to gain the approval of God.

In the entry on "Leprosy" in the *Medieval Disability Glossary*, Julie Orlemanski provides translations of two Middle English sermons that illustrate the range of reactions to leprosy. In one fourteenth-century sermon, there is what we might call a traditional model of leprosy that equates the disease with sin:

> For just as leprosy makes the body
> Ugly and loathsome and repulsive,
> So the filth of lechery makes
> The soul very loathsome spiritually,
> And the swelling of secret pride
> Is leprosy, which no man may hide. [69]

At the end of this passage is the central metaphor: that the symptoms of leprosy cannot be hidden, just as the spiritual symptoms of sin cannot be masked. There is an emphasis on words such as "ugly" and "loathsome," focusing on the physical manifestations of the disease. A fifteenth-century sermon presents leprosy differently, as a sign of blessing:

> There once lived a bishop in France who washed the feet of lepers. One day the bishop encountered a leper along the way. The bishop kissed him. The leper said, "Bishop, on account of your humility, wipe with your tongue out of my nose the snot that is hanging in there, because I cannot bear any linen cloth to touch it, it is so sore." The bishop with his tongue licked it out humbly. And in his licking, suddenly out of the leper's nose fell a precious stone into the bishop's mouth, shining bright and sweet-smelling. And then, in the sight of the bishop, the leper ascended up to heaven.[70]

---

68 Brenner, *Leprosy and Charity*, 1–2.

69 Hamilton, *The Leper King and His Heirs*, 254.

70 Translations of both texts from Orlemanski, "Leprosy."

Rather than a metaphor for sin, leprosy here is a positive spiritual opportunity, allowing the bishop to demonstrate his holiness through an act of humility. In addition, the leper proceeds to heaven, contradicting the earlier image of leprosy as sin. While these two texts are written in the same language within a century of each other, they demonstrate the range of representations of leprosy and thus the range of social perceptions.

Alexandra Houston explores this ambiguity as a development over time in "'Seiknes Incurabill': The Evolution of Literary Representations of Leprosy in Medieval and Early Modern English Narratives," in which she concludes that "the literature of the late medieval and early modern period shows a general trend away from a balance between suspicion and reverence that dominated the twelfth and thirteenth centuries toward a more cautious, hostile view."[71] Some of this evolution may be due to shifting ideas about disease due to the plague.

Perhaps no other figure better illustrates the contrasting view of lepers as social outcasts than Baldwin IV, the Leper King of Jerusalem from 1174 to 1185.[72] Despite being diagnosed with leprosy while his rule was still under the aegis of a regent, as he himself was too young at the age of thirteen, he ascended to the throne and was never fully segregated from others. Despite at times wanting to abdicate and amid the symptoms of his worsening condition, he fought in battles, negotiated political situations, and generally contributed to the well-being of his kingdom. It was the matter of his succession, as he could not marry and have children as a leper, that was of serious concern.

Leprosaria and the Mont-aux-Malades

Leprosaria were the first hospitals specializing in a disease.[73] The East Roman Empire opened leprosaria during the fourth century, the first being Sebasteia in central Asia Minor and the most famous outside of Constantinople.[74] In England, leprosaria were in use at least before 1100:

> the *leprosarium* at Harbledown was founded by Archbishop Lanfranc of Canterbury (1070–1089) in the 1080s, while recent excavations on the site of the leper house of St Mary Magdalen outside Winchester suggest that this

71 Houston, "'Seiknes Incurabill,'" 41.

72 See Hamilton, *The Leper King and His Heirs*.

73 See Wollina et al., "Leprosy in the Middle Ages."

74 Nesbitt and Miller, *Walking Corpses*, 72–75.

may have been an eleventh-century foundation, which could possibly have accommodated lepers before the Norman Conquest.[75]

In Jerusalem, by the 1140s, the Order of Saint Lazarus was "composed of knights and sergeants who had contracted leprosy, and who, as professed members of the Order, continued to fight as long as they were able to do so."[76] The Order was also in charge of the management of leper hospitals in the Kingdom.

Far from the isolated places of popular imagination, leprosaria often were connected to the communities around them, and, although many were in semi-rural areas due to a need for farmland and water supplies, they were generally "highly visible" and "situated along main roads."[77] The connection between lepers and charity translated to increased status and protection of their communities. Indeed, there is evidence of patronage for leprosaria from "bishops, emperors, wealthy private persons, and probably monasteries."[78] Those who gave such patronage "believed the foundation of such hospitals benefitted not only the lepers, whose sufferings paralleled those of the Son of God, but also their own spiritual purity."[79] In Robert Henryson's mid-fifteenth-century Scottish *Testament of Cresseid*, the main character, having developed leprosy, is depicted as "achieving repentance in the bequeathing of her earthly riches to the leprosarium."[80] Non-leprous individuals also at times decided to live in leprosaria in order to assist with the needs of the community or perhaps as repentance for their own sins.

Mont-aux-Malades was founded on a hill to the northwest of Rouen, France. Likely, it was originally a gathering of lepers that became institutionalized in the twelfth century. Receiving royal patronage, particularly after its rededication to Saint Thomas Becket in 1174 and becoming a focus for the charity of the local burgesses, their "gifts made the *leprosarium* community a significant property-owner within the city of Rouen, and thus linked it to the commercial and political activities of urban society."[81] While their location on a hill outside the city did correspond to Biblical instructions that lepers should be separated, it also provided an environment that was visible

75 Brenner, *Leprosy and Charity*, 20.

76 Hamilton, *The Leper King and His Heirs*, 29.

77 Brenner, *Leprosy and Charity*, 6, 20–21.

78 Nesbitt and Miller, *Walking Corpses*, 90.

79 Houston, "'Seiknes Incurabill,'" 31.

80 Houston, "'Seiknes Incurabill,'" 38.

81 Brenner, *Leprosy and Charity*, 20.

and one that was conducive to the care of lepers, given beliefs in the therapeutic benefits of fresh air.[82]

Leprosaria are communities in which those who experienced a common disease could live together and support each other. Their organized nature allowed for charity and patronage to benefit the inhabitants collectively rather than through begging or other individual methods of supporting themselves. It also benefited the supporters as a demonstration of spiritual well-being and in securing a ready-made community to pray on their behalf.

Contexts: The Language of Disability

Studying the language of disability in the Middle Ages is complex, both because of the many different languages used throughout the time and space of the global medieval period as well as in terms of the issues of translation.

It is nearly impossible to be expert in all of the languages necessary for widespread study of medieval disability. Even just in Europe, the issues of language create complexities and opportunities, and that deepens exponentially the more of the globe we cover. This fact demands collaboration among scholars working in different periods and geographies.

These issues become even more complicated, considering who has often produced translations of non-Western texts. An edition of *African Myths of Origin*, in which we can find references to disability, states that the "sources for the stories include European works published in the late nineteenth century, colonial era and modern accounts."[83] We can immediately see the problem in filtering indigenous texts through colonialist translation. Can we trust the translation? Can we make valuable analyses from the translation?

Another example is "A Woman Who Could Not Speak Is Healed, Owing to the Grace of the Kannon of Ishiyama" in the *Konjaku Monogatari Shu*. In the edition *Japanese Tales from Times Past: Stories of Fantasy and Folklore from the Konjaku Monogatari Shu*, one passage reads: "The nurse pitied her more and more, and grieved over her **handicap**...Although he still loved her, he came to visit her less frequently, because now he knew that she was **handicapped**."[84] In the Oxford English Dictionary, the word *handicap* is marked "Now offensive." United Access talks about the negative stereotypes of the word and how people with disabilities "rejected this term, recognizing the inherent biases it carried and the need for a more empowering and

---

82 Brenner, *Leprosy and Charity*, 21.

83 *African Myths of Origin*, ed. Belcher, 309.

84 *Japanese Tales from Times Past*, trans. Koriyama and Allen, 96. Emphases added.

respectful language."[85] Thus, when we read the words *handicap* and *handicapped* in this translation they automatically have negative associations, which may or may not have been intended in the original.

Case Study: Middle English *Wod* in Hagiography

Examining the appearances of the word *wod* in Middle English hagiography reveals that it is often a universal term for a variety of mental health symptoms, especially when it is allied with associations of anger, making it difficult to parse its exact meaning.

In the fifteenth-century *Sermon on St. Margaret* by John Mirk, he states that the saint's tormenter, Olibrius, is driven by the saint "mad for anger" (wode for wrothe): "But when she was brought before him, and he saw that she was of Christian faith, then he was mad for anger" (lines 30–32).[86] In the fifteenth-century *Stanzaic Life of Margaret*, it is stated that for "this glorious virgin his wits were near gone" (line 76), indicating that it is St. Margaret's beauty that is responsible for Olibrius' madness, intensified later on by her determination to remain faithful to her Christian faith. This could be dismissed, but his subsequent behaviour is extremely violent. In Mirk's *Sermon*:

> And because she would not give in to him, he had her hung up, and thus beat her with scourges, and razed her fair body with evils, that it was a wonder to see the great plenty of blood that came out of her body, and after had her cast in prison until the morrow, that he might think himself what was best to be done with her (lines 32–36).

John Mirk is consistent in his descriptions of such behaviour. For instance, in his *Sermon on St. Katherine*, there is a similar scene:

> Then anon Maxencius commanded to make a great, horrible fire and burn them all therein. But God showed here His miracle for them, so that there was no cloth they had nor any of their hair that had been touched with the fire, but all lay dead by each other with as fair an expression as if they had been asleep. Then was the Emperor mad for anger (wode for tene), and had Katherine stripped naked and thus beat her fair body with scourges, that all her fair body was full of wounds and running all with blood, and had her put in prison, to stay there thirty days without meat or drink until he came again (lines 40–49).

---

85 United Access, "History of the Term 'Handicapped.'"

86 All quotations from saints' lives of Margaret and the *Sermon on St. Katherine* are *Middle English Legends of Women Saints*, ed. Reames. Translations are mine. "Bot whan scheo was/broght beforyn hym, and he wyst that scheo was of Criston fayth, than was he/neygh wode for wrothe."

This time, the tormenter Maxencius is driven "mad for anger" (wode for tene) and then begins his torture of her. The use of *tene* here instead of Mirk's previous *wrothe* allows for some creative interpretation. The *Middle English Dictionary* definitions of *tene* range from "injury, harm, wrong" to "physical suffering pain; also the torment of hell," "hopelessness, despair," "vexation, chagrin; anger, wrath," and "a fit of anger, murderous rage." The example quotations provided in the entry that also reference *wod* are all included in the definition "vexation, chagrin; anger, wrath," which indeed would match the sense of the Margaret sermon. However, looking at this definition in context of the other possibilities, particularly "murderous rage" and "despair," reflects a particular sense of madness with a tendency towards a mental disorder.

Even when *wod* is not mentioned in Middle English texts, *wroth* (anger) is still common in the saints' lives. In the thirteenth or fourteenth-century *South English Legendary Martyrdom of St. Andrew*, the narrative of a male saint, the word appears three times in a short 108 lines, where it is used in reference to the tormenter Justice's reaction to the saint. When St. Andrew converts some of his people, the Justice is *wroth* (line 15).[87] Then he becomes so *wroth* that he throws Andrew in prison (line 51). Finally, the Justice's *wroth* causes him to order the torture of the saint—the kind that prevents the death of the tortured to increase the amount of pain and bloodshed (line 65).

The *South English Legendary Martyrdom of St. George*, another male saint, presents a visual description of the tormenter's reaction to the saint. Here, when St. George calls his tormenter's gods false, Dacian "grimaced and foamed fast" (grennede and femede vaste, line 15). This could, of course, be a metaphor for anger. "Foaming at the mouth" is, however, a very physical reaction that is frequently associated with mental health episodes. This image is increased as the text continues. As St. George's body is miraculously unharmed by the tortures Dacian orders, his anger grows: "Well angry (wroth) was Dacian when he saw this happen" (line 60). When boiling water does nothing to the saint—George even lies down and takes a nap—Dacian's "wit was nearly deprived of him" (wit him was nei bynome, line 73). From the initial image of a foaming mouth, we move to the declaration of the tormenter losing his wits as his increasingly violent tortures are ineffective.

---

87 All quotations from St. Andrew and St. George taken from *Saints' Lives in Middle English Collections*, ed. Whatley, Thompson, and Upchurch. Translations are mine.

Returning to female saints' lives, there is a similar image in John Capgrave's *Life of Saint Katherine*. As Katherine continues to defy his orders in the fifth and final book of the text, the emperor becomes mentally and visually agitated: "Now was the emperor almost mad and out of his mind: his eyes rolled as they would fall out" (Now wax the emperour ny wode and oute of mynde:/His eyne rolled as thei wold fall oute, V.155–56). The internal description of going "mad" and "out of his mind" is accompanied by the external sign of eyes rolling, as if they would fall out of his head. This description is followed by the emperor ordering the death by fire of all the people Katherine has managed to convert with her speeches. He says at this point that he will not eat or drink until he sees them "burned and stinking." The emperor is later described in typical fashion as "mad for anger" (wode for ire, V.603). This madness is not only depicted in the one tormenter, but also by others of his employ, emphasizing its presence in the text. In book four of the saint's life, a Master Astenes rises to speak his anger at the saint's continued resistance. His "haughty disposition" (fers corage, IV.1404) is described as "madness" (wodeness) and then he is attributed with "anger of choler" (angyr of coloure, IV.1406). At the end of the text, when Katherine is beheaded, her executioner "was glad to do the command of his lord" (was glad to do the comaundment/Of his lord, V.1890–91), and then "with a stroke that was full of madness and rage her head he parted from her body there" (with a stroke that was ful wode and rage / Hir hede he parted from hir body there, V.1895–96). An extension of the emperor, the very stroke that takes the saint's life is described as being *ful wode and rage.*

Capgrave's text also provides us with a secondary yet important character who characterizes the emperor's actions in terms of madness. His own queen, converted to Christianity, confronts her husband as the tortures of the saint increase. She says to him:

> You, wretched husband, what have you done?
> Why do you torment so wrongly this good maid?
> Against the great God why do you wrestle so?
> What madness (wodnes) makes you with care and woe
> To pursue God's servants with pain and death? (IV.1423–27)

The queen very deliberately calls the emperor's actions against the saint "madness" (wodnes). Her moment of resistance is met with equal violence from her husband, as he has her breasts pulled off, her body beaten, and her head cut off, all in his own sight, confirming that his violence is not just aimed at Katherine but also his own family, and especially women.

Providing an interesting point of contrast, the fifteenth-century English *Life of Mary of Oegines* does not have a tormenter at the level of these previous ones, but she is castigated for her excessive weeping, especially by one particular priest. The saint asks of God that the priest would be shown that her weeping was not in her control:

> Wherefore that priest, while he sang mass that same day, was so overcome with abundance of tears, that his spirit was well-nigh strangled; and the more that he busied him to refrain his tears, the more not only he but also the skin and the outer clothes were wet with water of weeping: so he that ill-advised, he that put blame on Christ's maiden, learned with shame by experience what he should do that he would not first know by meekness and compassion.[88]

Here, Mary's tormenter-priest's "spirit was well-nigh strangled." More significant is that the priest "learned with shame by experience" what he did not at first treat with "meekness and compassion." Through his experience of the uncontrollable weeping, the priest is able to empathize with Mary's experience. The tormenter's behaviour in attempting to humiliate Mary should certainly not be dismissed, but this behaviour is more commensurate with standard anger, frustration, and contempt, emphasizing the extreme difference in the reactions of tormentors in the previous texts—ones that use specific language to describe them.

These various usages of the Middle English word *wod* demonstrate the necessity for interpretation when considering medieval words for disability.

88 Translation is mine and Alicia Protze's, taken from Horstmann, "Prosalegenden."

Chapter 3

MAKING THE INTANGIBLE TANGIBLE

IN THIS SECTION of the exhibition, we could imagine a voice filtering through the speakers and surrounding us, as a storyteller begins a tale.

Section 1: Mental Health

If physical disability lacks representation in heritage spaces, mental disability has even less representation. Through the study of trauma in museums as well as how medieval disability in general is represented in these spaces, it becomes clear that historical mental disability is marginalized. There are many reasons for this. One is the lingering stigma of mental health issues and a general reluctance to engage with related subjects. Another is the difficulty in analyzing mental disability in historical contexts, especially in time periods prior to psychoanalysis and its terminology. A significant barrier is how to depict what are often intangible disabilities in a physical manner. Acquiescing to these limitations has the consequence of erasing people with mental disabilities from history, which is both a misrepresentation of the past and damaging to modern peoples.

Looking at the mental health word "depression" in different versions of English can demonstrate the complexity of the numerous medieval words related to mental health with their respective meanings in many languages. The Old English (OE) word *un-mód* is defined in Bosworth and Toller's Anglo-Saxon Dictionary as "despondency, dejection."[1] The quotation offered in Bosworth-Toller for *un-mód* is taken from the *Leechdoms*, edited by Cockayne. As the title notes, this is a work focused on Old English documentation of medical knowledge, and the section including this word discusses the symptoms of stomach diseases. In Cockayne's edition, *un-mód* is translated to "despondency" and is followed by *ungemetwæccum* (excessive wakefulness). A second OE term *mód-leást* translates to "despondency." *Mód-leást* has a clear meaning in Aelfric's *Lives of Saints* in his account of the life of St. Agnes (here, from Skeat's edition):

1 See the Bosworth and Toller Dictionary at https://bosworthtoller.com/.

DOI: 10.17302/asgs32687 © Arc Humanities Press

> The youth was angered, and inwardly blinded
> after the maiden's speech, who had spurned him with words.
> He straightaway fell ill, and drew sighs
> from the depths of his breast, lying on his bed.
> Then leeches enquired why he was lying there,
> and made known to the father the youth's **mental disorder**
> (***mód-leáste***) (lines 63–68).[2]

Skeat's translation of *mód-leáste* to "mental disorder" is itself a statement upon the word. The youth in question is in particular suffering from love-sickness (or at least from his offer of marriage being rejected), which connects it with a typical use in the Anglo-Norman of the word *pensif*. Here, the youth exhibits symptoms such as falling ill, sighing, being confined to bed. His malady requires attention from doctors.

The Middle English (ME) word *dēpressiŏun* has three definitions in the Middle English Dictionary, the second of which is "(b) lowering of spirits, dejection."[3] Following from that definition, the ME word *dējecciŏun* is defined as "depression of spirits, despondency." The ME word *grẹvŏushēde* is defined as "melancholy, depression." The ME word *langŏur* poses more complicated issues. It can be defined in a variety of ways. The definitions that apply here include: "sickness," "disease," "physical affliction, "infirmity," "misery," "physical or mental suffering," "anguish," "depression," "self-disgust."

The example given in the Middle English Dictionary for *dēpressiŏun* is the text of *Life of Mary of Oegines*, which portrays St. Mary with a variety of mental health indicators, in particular fluctuating mental states, issues with food, and self-violence. Indeed, Mary characterizes her relationship to God and her faith in terms of depression:

> And when she prayed specially for anybody, as with a wonderful experience our Lord showed to her and answered her spirit. Truly, she perceived meanwhile by elation of her spirit or depression whether she were heard or not.[4]

For Mary, it is through "elation of her spirit or depression" that she is able to gauge the success of her communication with God. In outward signs of intangible disability, the saint also frequently cries uncontrollably, and yet this experience too is couched in terms of a positive relationship with God. Her fasting, even to the point of potential eating disorders, as well as the

---

2 *Aelfric's Lives of Saints*, ed. and trans. Skeat.

3 See the Middle English Dictionary at https://quod.lib.umich.edu/m/middle-english-dictionary/dictionary.

4 Translation is mine and Alicia Protze's, taken from Horstmann, "Prosalegenden."

cutting of her own skin, are also represented as natural manifestations of her sainthood.

This look at one mental health term highlights the difficulties in giving form to intangible heritage; yet, while historical mental disability can be elusive, it is not impossible to imagine.

The Peacemaker and the Tadadaho

Oral Story; Haudenosaunee, Northeastern North America, eleventh to fifteenth centuries[5]

A rich source for studying medieval disability is oral storytelling. In speaking about studying premodern disability in Africa, Magnus Mfoafo-M'Carthy, Jeff Grischow, and Festus Moasun comment:

> It is very difficult to reconstruct the history of disability in precolonial Africa, let alone the territory that became Ghana. Written sources are limited to Muslim chronicles beginning in the thirteenth century and European travelers' accounts in the 1700s and 1800s...Beyond these sources, there also exist oral traditions and proverbs that can be mined for information about the history of disability. In some cases, this material can be accessed in written form, but researchers also must rely on the accounts of contemporary fieldwork participants who are familiar with traditions surrounding disability.[6]

Representations of disability are not always overt and, at times, require scholars to interpret sources, including these oral traditions. Such an example is the story of the Peacemaker and the Tadadaho, which is set during the creation of the Haudenosaunee Confederacy. It is unclear exactly when the Confederacy was formed, but it was pre-European contact in North America, likely mid-fifteenth century or even possibly earlier.

The Story of the Peacemaker and the Tadadaho

This summary of the story of the Peacemaker and the Tadadaho is based on the version told for Tree Media by storyteller Chief Oren Lyons, Faithkeeper of the Turtle Clan of the Onondaga Nation.

---

5 I was introduced to this story by Dr. Hilary Weaver, Professor Emeritus of Social Work at the University at Buffalo School of Social Work and Lakota, who has lived much of her adult life in Haudenosaunee territory in Western New York; she explained that it is beginning to be looked at through the mental health lens by some indigenous scholars and storytellers.

6 Mfoafo-M'Carthy, Grischow, and Moasun, *Experiencing Disability Stigma*, 17.

During the time when the Peacemaker was attempting to form the Haudenosaunee Confederacy, he brought together four of the great nations to lay out his plan for peace. He wanted to include the fifth nation, and he had to seek out its Tadadaho, or leader. Unfortunately, the Tadadaho lived deep in the swamp by himself. He was "fierce," "almost unrecognizable as a human" with "snakes in his hair." He seemed to have little need or desire to join the Confederacy and rejected any attempts to reach him.

When the Peacemaker first travelled to the Mohawk shore of the Onondaga Lake, he spent the night at a lodge nearby owned by a woman, Jigonhsasee. She was inspired by his peace plan, and she agreed to help in any way that she could, especially in talking with the people who would travel by and stay with her.

When the Tadadaho refused to listen to the Peacemaker, he sent for the woman. After she arrived, they asked if she could help, and she explained that she had been hearing a song over and over again in her head. She taught the song to the Peacemaker and his men, and they began to sing it.

The Tadadaho was drawn to the song "against his will" until they could speak to him. At first, he was still resistant to their arguments, but the more he listened, the more they could see "the snakes falling from his hair," as he began to "transform." They promised him that, if he joined the Confederacy, he would be its leader and the title of "Tadadaho" would prevail, to which he agreed.

After that, the Peacemaker planted a tree of peace, setting symbolic animals in its branches, and asked the nations to throw away their weapons, cementing the Confederacy.

The Medusa Effect

Reading the story of the Peacemaker and the Tadadaho from a disability perspective reveals intriguing aspects of mental health. In this version told by Chief Lyons, there is a strong emphasis placed on the Tadadaho removing himself from the community and living in the swamp. He is described as "almost unrecognizable as a human" with "snakes in his hair." The former indicates that his physical features reflect some inner turmoil. Indeed, Lesli J. Favor, in a primary source investigation of *The Iroquois Constitution*, describes him as a "misshapen monster."[7] In the version from *The Iroquois Book of Rites* published in 1883, his very name means "entangled," and,

---

7 Favor, *The Iroquois Constitution*, 20.

instead of simply being on his head, the snakes replace his hair and are described as "writhing."[8]

The snakes are a key element in a mental health reading. While on one hand they can represent a physically monstrous figure, they seem rather to represent the Tadadaho's mental state. Half a world away and several centuries removed, another story famously uses snakes in a character's hair as a sign of the trauma she endures. As narrated by Roman poet Ovid in Book 4 of the *Metamorphoses* (first century CE), Medusa was a beautiful woman raped by the god Neptune in the goddess Minerva's temple—both a criminal and blasphemous act. Minerva punishes Medusa by turning her into a monster living isolated from others with snakes for hair and the ability to turn men to stone with her gaze. There has been much scholarly discussion of this story in terms of the seeming punishment of the woman rather than the rapist as well as the metaphoric meaning of Medusa's appearance and her subsequent life as a monster. In thinking of the woman as a rape victim, her trauma and anger at what she experienced is understandable. The hissing snakes that replaced her hair, which Ovid writes was previously considered her most beautiful feature, drawing Neptune's attention and lust, are a fitting representation of her mental health. Unfortunately, the snakes remain in place until she is decapitated by Perseus without any opportunity for Medusa to work through her trauma.

The Tadadaho, conversely, is given that opportunity. After being soothed by Jigonhsasee's song, the snakes fall out of his hair, indicating a transformation that allows him both to listen to the Peacemaker and to rejoin the community he had previously isolated himself from. In addition, it is important to note here that the community he is reentering is one that is committing itself to peace.

Music Therapy

Another aspect of the Tadadaho story to emphasize is the song that soothes him. Jigonhsasee's song, introduced to her naturally by the birds near her home, has the effect of calming the Tadadaho to the point he is able to listen. Chief Lyons describes it as drawing him out "against his will," indicating that he fought against it. Metaphorically, this is a representation both of the difficult process of therapy of any kind and, more specifically, of the effects of music therapy.

8 *The Iroquois Book of Rites*. This version presents a far more sinister version of Tadadaho, but is also edited by a non-indigenous editor.

Music as therapy is not a new concept. Michael H. Thaut finds that it is "based on ancient cross-cultural beliefs that music can have a 'healing' effect on mind and body," and he provides examples from "preliterate cultures," "early civilizations," "antiquity, with an emphasis on Greek writings on music and medicine," and the "Middle Ages, Renaissance, and Baroque, with treatises on music for therapeutic purposes."[9] In *Music as Medicine*, Peregrine Horden claims, "At various times and in various cultures over the past two and a half millennia—and probably still further back in time—music has been medicine. Performing or listening to music...maintains or restores the health of mind, and even, body."[10] A prominent ancient example is in the biblical account of David, who is represented as soothing King Saul's mental torment with music (1 Samuel 16:14–23). According to Horden's work, understanding of the therapeutic qualities of music seems to be a near-universal constant across culture and geography. Referring to medieval Europe, Christopher Callahan states, "In its most cherished formative texts, both secular and sacred, the medieval world encountered the notion that music had measurable therapeutic value."[11] Speaking generally, Erin Suzanne Fly comments that, throughout time, Native American peoples have perceived music "as a powerful tool for medicinal and community uses, and have seen it as essential in everyday life."[12] Music therapy as a profession with certifications and training may be a more modern concept, but its roots are ancient.

Oral Storytelling

One of the issues of studying historical disability is the different types of sources that need to be consulted or collected in addition to the traditional written records, which have been privileged for far too long. Premodern indigenous sources tend to be oral traditions. In terms of heritage, the international Convention for the Safeguarding of the Intangible Cultural Heritage, adopted by UNESCO in 2003, provides a definition of intangible cultural heritage that includes "oral traditions and expressions, including language as a vehicle of the intangible cultural heritage."[13] *American Writers, Supplement XXVI*, a collection of literary biographical articles, includes Deganawida, the

---

9 Thaut, "Music as Therapy," 143.

10 Horden, *Music as Medicine*, 1.

11 Callahan, "Music in Medieval Medical Practice," 151.

12 Fly, "Multicultural Music Therapy," 19.

13 See the Convention for the Safeguarding of the Intangible Cultural Heritage, article 2(2)(a).

Peacemaker, as an author. In his article in that volume, Christopher Buck argues that Deganawida's stories should be considered "orature" (a blend of "oral" and "literature") that should be "recognized as part of the American literary canon" and, further, Deganawida was "a *maker* of history and culture, long before American literati came on the scene."[14] It does raise questions considering the dating of these sources and how or if we need to define a "definitive" version, such as reconciling the different retellings of the Peacemaker and the Tadadaho. These questions, however, are common ones with which medieval scholars engage.

"Mad" Henry of Fordwich Stained Glass

Canterbury Cathedral, England, late twelfth to thirteenth centuries

The stained-glass windows at Canterbury Cathedral are famous depictions of biblical stories, saints, and royal figures, and the life and miracles of St. Thomas Becket—the archbishop who was murdered in the cathedral in 1170. The Cathedral is well known for its central role in Geoffrey Chaucer's fourteenth-century masterpiece, the *Canterbury Tales*. The windows are survivors, having lived through, with some later repairs and replacements, the Reformation and World War II. They survived the latter only because of the foresight taken to remove them and place them in storage at the beginning of the War.[15]

The miracle windows surround the shrine to St. Thomas in the Trinity chapel, most taken from Benedict of Peterborough's *Miracles*. Benedict was a contemporary and biographer of Becket. Many of the stories depicted in these windows relate to disability. In window nV, William (the priest) is cured of a paralysis of the tongue. Goditha, in window nIV, is able to walk again after being unable to support herself on swollen feet. Other panels in nIV present William of Dene and the paralysis of his lower body and Richard of Stanley's contracted fingers. Goditha of Hayes is cured of dropsy in window nIII, as is the lameness of the two daughters of Godbold of Boxley and the leprosy of Ralph of Longueville. Also depicted in nIII is Eilward, who miraculously was allowed to see again despite his eyes having been gouged out. These are but some of the stories of physical disability told in the miracle windows.

14 Buck, "Deganawida, the Peacemaker," 82.

15 Dean and Chapter of Canterbury Cathedral, "Stained Glass in Canterbury Cathedral."

Other windows narrate stories of mental disability. One in particular is that of Henry of Fordwich.

The Story of Henry of Fordwich

The story of Henry of Fordwich is recorded in the miracles of St. Thomas by Benedict:

> What is easier—to give health to the mind or to the body? The one who illuminated the eyes of this man's body also restored the mind of Henry, a youth from Fordwich. He had been insane for several days and had inflicted on his friends an unexpected wound of pain. His hands were tied behind his back and he was dragged to the saint. Though he resisted and cried out, he was presented to the saint. All that day he remained insane, and then, as the light of the sun receded, he began gradually to recover the light of rationality. He spent the night in the church and left the next day in most perfect health (II.13).[16]

This tale is visually represented in two round panels in window nIV. On the left one, an individual, Henry, is bent over, clearly agitated, with his hands tied behind his back. Two others, the friends from Benedict's version, are on either side dragging Henry, while one has a raised stick, as if to beat him. A monk watches them from behind the shrine of Becket with one hand on a Bible. At the top of the scene are the Latin words *AMENS ACCEDIT*, or "the insane person approaches." In the second panel, on the right, Henry is calm and kneeling, his hands untied as they are clasped in prayer. The two friends stand beside him, one with hands in prayer as well while the other seems to be gesturing in amazement. The monk has a hand to his forehead, as if also marveling at what he has seen. The Latin inscription at the top of this panel is *ORAT SANUSQUE RECEDIT*, or "he prays and is healed and leaves." The rope used to bind Henry and the sticks used to beat him are at the base of the panel.

Although short, Henry's story is filled with information. We have a young man who seemingly abruptly starts to act differently than usual, even acting violently, and wounds his friends. Benedict often equates erratic behaviour with "madness," even when that behaviour is the result of healing. He says of Edmund, who was blind in one eye and received a drop of the saint's blood in it, that, when the healing began, he fell face-first to the ground and "twisted about, shouting" and that "you would have thought him to be insane as the

---

16 Benedict of Peterborough, *The Passion and Miracles of St. Thomas Becket*, ed. Koopmans, 120–21.

divine power healed him" (II.9).[17] Henry's friends' reaction is worth noting, as it differs between the textual and the visual versions. In Benedict's text, they drag him, bound, as he resists, to the shrine of Becket. This also seems to be the case in the window. However, in the stained glass, one of the friends appears to be beating him. This is far more extreme. One more element that appears in the window and not in the text is the monk bystander. His presence lends credence to the scene as he acts as witness to the miracle.

Binding Henry can, perhaps, be justified, given his violent behaviour; the fact that the friends take him to the saint rather than to an authority of the law or a prison, indicates that they are hoping to help him. Benedict does indicate in other miracles that those exhibiting such behaviour might be chained more seriously. In the story of William Patrick, who was in such pain from a toothache that his "cries and gestures" seemed like he was "mad rather than in pain," Benedict opines that without divine interference he might "have been placed in [the hardness of] chains as a madman" (I.14).[18] Benedict also seems to approve of the care of such individuals by family and friends; in the story of Walter of Grimsby of "unsound mind," "his friends and relatives procured his health for him from the martyr," although it seems only their vow to take him to Saint Thomas was enough rather than binding him (IV.57).[19] The visual depiction of Henry's beating, however, is far less justified. Henry is already bound, and there are two of them to contain him. Beating him as well seems excessive, and the fact that it is not in the source material raises questions. Here, the stories align again as Henry recovers. According to the Canterbury Historical and Archaeological Society's analysis of this window, the rope and sticks in the second panel are "left as an 'ex voto,' a thanks offering."[20] Such a reading is curious: why would the saint want these items representing violence as signs of gratitude? They are, however, no longer necessary after Henry is healed, and so perhaps the representation of their discarding is more symbolic than devotional.

17 Benedict of Peterborough, *The Passion and Miracles of St. Thomas Becket*, ed. Koopmans, 118.

18 Benedict of Peterborough, *The Passion and Miracles of St. Thomas Becket*, ed. Koopmans, 99–100.

19 Benedict of Peterborough, *The Passion and Miracles of St. Thomas Becket*, ed. Koopmans, 266.

20 Canterbury Historical and Archaeological Society, "Miracle Windows North Aisle."

A Parallel Literary Story

Parallel stories to Henry's exist in other saints' lives. In the late Middle English *Shorter South English Legendary Life of St. Frideswide*, there is a scene in which Frideswide encounters an individual very similar to Henry (lines 96–111).[21] A fisherman, sleeping amongst his friends in a boat, suddenly begins to display erratic behaviour. He, too, inflicts wounds on his companions, gnawing on them. They bind him, although there is no indication that they harm him in any other way, and they take him directly to St. Frideswide—again, not to any legal authority. In this story, the saint interacts directly with the fisherman, forming the sign of the cross on his head. This action causes the man to faint. Frideswide unbinds him and tells him to arise, which he does "whole and sound."

Access to the Holy

There is another story about Becket, as told by Benedict, with connections to mental health. Elward of Selling is described as hallucinating and being not in his "right mind":

> A certain man from Selling of adult age and large stature, Elward by name, had gone insane. Wherever he turned, he thought the enemy of the human race confronted him. He ordered him to be gone in the name of the Lord and spat as if spitting into his face. He was led to the saint and placed next to the sepulchre, and there he saw that diabolical phantom that seemed to be striking him. Not knowing where to turn, he fled to the martyr, and in a wonderful way he thrust his whole body through the narrow aperture that was hardly able to admit a human head. Without any difficulty, he wound himself inside this very narrow space in such a way that his head was at the martyr's feet and his feet at the martyr's head. Once he was stretched out upon the body of the saint in this way, he became quiet for a little while. We became concerned about how he would get out, and thought that the structure would definitely have to be broken apart for him to exit. Beyond all expectation, he came out of the other opening. Later, when he was in his right mind, we ordered him to go inside again. No matter how hard he tried, he could not get his shoulders into the aperture, not even with his clothes off. We made an adolescent with a thin and boyish body also try to do it, and we saw that his attempts were useless (II.31).[22]

---

21 *Middle English Legends of Women Saints*, ed. Reames.

22 Benedict of Peterborough, *The Passion and Miracles of St. Thomas Becket*, ed. Koopmans, 134.

Once again, we have the individual's companions taking him to the shrine of St. Thomas, here with no mention of violence. Frightened by his own hallucinations, Elward manages to push himself through the grating surrounding the saint's body and lies down next to it, which seems to soothe him into sleep. This is presented by Benedict as a miracle, for no one could fit through the grating, and Elward is described as being even larger than most people. After Elward is healed, they try to get him to repeat the incident, but to no avail. They even try to have a young boy squeeze through the opening, also without success. In addition to emphasizing that this act was a miracle of the saint, it is interesting that it is only when he is "mad" that Elward is allowed to approach the saint's body so closely. Once he is healed, he is no longer given that privilege.

The two versions of Henry of Fordwich's story—both the textual and its visual, stained-glass retelling—are rich sources of information about representations of mental disability. They tell us that medieval people were aware of its existence and sought remedies, which, in these cases, were spiritual or divine ones. Reactions to erratic or atypical behaviour varied from compassionate to violent, particularly depending on whether or not the individuals were a danger to themselves or others.

Stories: Wandering in the Saint Clare Garden

Santa Clara University, California, 2003

Another way to examine understandings of disability is by looking at methods of healing. We will sometimes see people with disabilities (or others on their behalf) seeking healing as a cure or for alleviation of symptoms, making examination of methods of healing particularly useful.

In terms of mental health, the methods of healing are varied, even within the same continent. For example, in West African countries, the *ndeup* is a community ritual performed in premodern and modern times to alleviate an array of psychological conditions, such as depression and trauma.[23] The *putchu guinadji* are figures carrying a shield on horseback, originating from the Kotoko people of Cameroon and Chad; they are intended to help their carriers with mental health issues.[24] Ethiopian *däbtäras* are unordained clerics who practise traditional medicine. They can create healing scrolls: "Healing scrolls are written in Ge'ez, a 2,000-year-old indigenous Semitic

23 See Solomon, *The Noonday Demon.*

24 See Christoph, "The Secret of the Putchu Guinadji."

language...Ethiopian magical literature—which includes healing scrolls—relies upon the invocation of the secret names of god (asmat). By mastering these many names, a däbtära or other priest can oblige God to aid his client. The scrolls' prayers are composed of passages from Christian books that invoke these or other protective and curative words."[25] These are only a few examples from various areas in Africa.

Natural remedies, derived from plants or other biological material, were commonly used to create healing methods for many diseases, disabilities, and even everyday ailments. Several of the recipes that have survived have been found to be far more effective than one might think based on a Westernized,modern understanding of medicine.[26] Medieval gardens were a typical location to find the ingredients for these remedies.

In 2003, Santa Clara University in California created a garden memorial to St. Clare of Assisi, who lived approximately 1193–1253. She was one of the first followers of St. Francis of Assisi and founded the Franciscan Order of Poor Ladies. The Mission Santa Clara was founded in 1777 by Spanish missionaries, which ultimately led to the naming of the city of Santa Clara and, subsequently, the university, with the latter being built around the Mission. It is worth noting that the Mission was the first in California to be named after a female saint.[27] The garden was founded on the 750th anniversary of Clare's death.

The Saint Clare Garden is designed to combine characteristics of typical medieval monastic gardens. It is organized into five sections, representing different stages of Clare's life. The Wild Flowers symbolize her childhood, growing up in Italy. The Medicinal and Household Herbs are part of her young adulthood, during which she learned how to run a noble house in preparation for marriage. The Lavender Garden, which surrounds a basin representing baptism, symbolizes her conversion at age nineteen. The Kitchen Garden contains plants that would have been cultivated at her monastery at San Damiano. The Mary Garden is made of plants that would have been found in southern and western Europe in the thirteenth century, with names connecting them to Mary, Christ, and the saints.[28]

The Medicinal and Household Herbs section is where many of the plants used in natural remedies are found. They include trees, shrubs, and vines;

25 Windmuller-Luna, "Ethiopian Healing Scrolls."

26 See, for example, Rayner, "AncientBiotics."

27 California Missions Foundation, "History of Mission Santa Clara de Asís."

28 Lucid, "St. Clare Garden."

groundcovers, herbs, and perennials; and annuals. Among these are rosemary, also known as Mary's Tree, and sage, known as Mary's Shawl.[29]

According to the *Zibaldone da Canal*, written by a Venetian merchant in the fourteenth century, rosemary could be used to treat symptoms commonly associated with mental health issues: "Likewise, take the leaves of the rosemary and put it in your bed, and you will not have nightmares.... Likewise, take the leaf of the rosemary, and boil it, and wash your head, and great weakness from rage, or other causes, will fall away from you, and you will be well."[30] Similarly, in the 1525 *Banckes's Herbal*, the first printed English herbal, which was based on the mid-fourteenth century "On the Virtues of Rosemary" (created for the Countess of Hainault Jeanne de Valoise), rosemary has similar characteristics: "Take the flowers thereof and make powder thereof and binde it to thy right arme in a linnen cloath and it shale make thee light and merrie.... Also put the leaves under thy bedde and thou shalt be delivered of all evill dreames."[31] Nightmares, or evil dreams, can be a sign of mental distress, particularly caused by traumatic events. Rage is another potential sign, especially when it causes physical weakness, and needing a remedy to "make you light and merry" may be an indication of experiencing depression. Another well-known printed herbal, *The Grete Herball*, from the sixteenth century, which was a translation of an earlier text, the French *Le Grant Herbier* (1498), which itself took heavily from the *Circa instans*, a work from Salerno, Italy (mid-twelfth century) that describes treatment with rosemary for the alleviation of "weyknesse of ye brayne."[32] This description could cover a wide variety of mental issues. Sage is also described as having mental health benefits. In the *Tacuinum sanitatis*, originally an eleventh-century Arabic medical treatise later translated into Latin, sage is described as being able to calm the nerves, which could indicate a treatment for the symptoms of anxiety.[33]

A walk through the Saint Clare Garden, particularly the Medicinal and Household Herbs section, is a link to medieval natural remedies and, in particular, those that were used to address mental health symptoms. And a walk through a garden is often cited as therapeutic in itself.

---

29 Lucid, "Medicinal Plant List for the St. Clare Garden."

30 *Merchant Culture in Fourteenth-Century Venice*, ed. Dotson, 149–51.

31 Rohde, *The Old English Herbals.*

32 Rohde, *The Old English Herbals.*

33 Arano, *The Medieval Health Handbook.*

Section 2: Trauma

The link between disability and trauma is, at the least, two-fold: one, disabilities stemming from trauma, such as post-traumatic stress disorder (PTSD), and, two, trauma experienced by the disabled, such as abuse or the consequences of social perception.

Recent discussions and events have centred on the trauma that can be caused by cultural heritage—most notably exposure to the Confederate monuments in the United States—and the trauma that can be healed by it, such as memorials designed and poetry written after the Boston Marathon bombings.[34] This discussion reaches back into the premodern, with the toppling of monuments to despotic kings or the erection of memorials to grief, such as the Eleanor crosses in England, providing insight into how cultural heritage can both incite and heal trauma.

Towton Head 25

Skull; Battle of Towton, England, 1461

The Battle of Towton was an encounter in the Wars of the Roses that took place on March 29, 1461, during a snowstorm in Yorkshire, England. It is considered to be potentially the largest and bloodiest battle fought on English soil, with around 28,000 casualties.[35] In terms of medieval battles, it is an extreme representation of the violence and trauma of war.

In 1996, construction at Towton Hall revealed an unexpected discovery: the mass grave of individuals who had died in this battle. The Towton Battlefield Archaeology Project states that there were the remains of approximately fifty individuals in the grave, and "all individuals were males who had suffered extensive trauma, inflicted by swords, knives, bills, and war hammers."[36] Information from this discovery brought to light the "human cost of medieval warfare."[37] It also serves as evidence of the physical trauma of battle and a starting point for considering the psychological trauma as well.

---

34 See *Displaced Heritage.*

35 See Historic UK's "The Battle of Towton" site.

36 Sutherland, "Introduction."

37 Fiorato, "The Context of the Discovery," 2.

The Story of Towton Head 25

In Shannon A. Novak's review of the "battle-related trauma" evidenced by the remains in the Towton mass grave, she assesses that they are the result of "hand-to-hand combat in a brutal battle using very efficient weapons of war."[38] She concludes, "If the skeletons from this mass grave attest to at least a facet of the battle, these men died in a frenzied killing that involved numerous blows to the head, often after they were incapacitated and unable to defend themselves."[39] Novak questions how effective and what usage there was of helmets in this battle, given the "the level of head trauma."[40]

One skull in particular, known as Towton Head 25, tells a bloody story. So bloody that it warranted its own discussion in Novak's review:

> Eight distinct wounds, all from blades, affected the head...this may not have been the first battle in which this individual participated. Evidence of a well-healed depression fracture occurs in the left parietel. A series of three blade skip marks skirt the bone along the left frontal. Two small nicks also appear on the left side of the mandible. A deeper penetrating wound occurs in the left parietal.... These five wounds most likely occurred during face-to-face attack by a right handed assailant wielding a bladed instrument.... A large horizontal blade would bisects the occipital bone and deeply penetrates the endocranium.... Large flakes of bone bend internally to the point of impact and would have resulted in extensive trauma to the brain. This blow [delivered from the back with a large bladed instrument] would have certainly incapacitated this individual and was most likely lethal...After this individual was brought down and presumably dead, two more injuries occurred... The blade wound resulted in the face being bisected and at such a depth that the entire palate was also bisected internally.[41]

The Bosworth Battlefield Heritage Centre displays a panel highlighting Towton Head 25 to illustrate the brutality of war as well as medical treatments for war wounds. They emphasize that this individual had likely lost use of the left side of his face due to the earlier wound that had healed, which had nearly cut off his jaw.[42] This person had survived a serious, disfiguring injury in a previous battle only to succumb to his wounds at the Battle of Towton. It is important to highlight in Novak's assessment the amount of physical trauma to the brain that this individual sustained. We have to think

38 Novak, "Battle-Related Trauma," 101.

39 Novak, "Battle-Related Trauma," 101.

40 Novak, "Battle-Related Trauma," 101.

41 Novak, "Battle-Related Trauma," 100.

42 This panel was available in the Heritage Centre in 2016.

about the results of that trauma, had he survived, and how others who certainly did survive experienced their trauma in and following this and other battles.

The Case of Henry VIII

The story of an infamous name in history can potentially shed more light on the effects of brain trauma inflicted in war. Muhammad Qaiser Ikram, Fazle Hakim Sajjad, and Arash Salardini find that King Henry VIII of England, who lived from 1491–1547, suffered at various times from amnesia, impulse control, sociopathy, depression, headaches, and insomnia, and they associate these symptoms with traumatic brain injury as a result of his sporting activities.[43] Sport jousting, while not an activity of war, was intended to mimic the battlefield and resulted in similar injuries—even at times mortal ones. Indeed, "Henry was knocked off his horse while jousting in January of 1536.... His fully armored horse fell on top of him, rendering him unconscious for some two hours. The longer the period of unconsciousness, the greater and more lasting the brain injury tends to be. His legs may have been broken in the fall, as well."[44] The king is notorious for his erratic behaviour later in life, and these researchers postulate that his jousting injuries—particularly one in 1536—are partially responsible for this behaviour. Along with the physical symptoms of traumatic brain injury, the National Institute of Neurological Disorders and Stroke notes cognitive or psychological symptoms as well, including mood swings, agitation, anxiety, depression, confusion, disorientation, memory problems, frustration, and irritability.[45] It is also noted that traumatic brain injury can co-exist with PTSD, because brain injuries are often sustained in traumatic experiences.[46]

The Life of a Medieval Soldier

The Book of Chivalry by Geoffroi de Charny, written in the fourteenth century, is a treatise about how to be a good knight and warrior, identifying both desirable and undesirable behaviours. Geoffroi does indicate that being a soldier is not a glamorous life, and it comes with many hardships:

---

43 Ikram, Sajjad, and Salardini, "The Head That Wears the Crown."

44 Waugaman, "Traumatic Brain Injury," 374.

45 National Institute of Neurological Disorders and Stroke, "Traumatic Brain Injury (TBI)."

46 See Bryant, "Post-Traumatic Stress Disorder."

> For, whoever might want to consider the hardships, pains, discomforts, fears, perils, broken bones, and wounds which the good knights who uphold the order of knighthood as they should endure and have to suffer frequently, there is no religious order in which as much is suffered as has to be endured by these good knights who go in search of deeds of arms in the right way as has been set forth above.[47]

While mostly focusing on the physical with "broken bones" and "wounds," he also lists "fears" and "perils." He elaborates at one point on this emotional toll:

> We therefore learn from the good knights and men-at-arms whose great achievements and honorable deeds of prowess and of valor have been related, described, and told above and which they have accomplished through suffering great hardship, making strenuous efforts, and enduring fearful physical perils and the loss of friends whose deaths they have witnessed in many great battles in which they have taken part; these experiences have often filled their hearts with great distress and strong emotion.[48]

While not a clinical description of PTSD, the final line about "great distress and strong emotion" is a testimony to the lingering psychological effects of witnessing and participating in warfare, especially for those for whom the military is a profession or a long-standing experience.

Towton Head 25 is a tragic reminder of the traumatic experiences of soldiers, both medieval and present-day. Undergoing injuries of this nature and watching others receive such wounds have long-term physical and psychological consequences.

The Magdeburg Black Madonna

Wood Statue; Magdeburg Cathedral, Germany, Thirteenth Century

Representations of the Virgin Mary, especially in the Middle Ages, are vast and, although demonstrating patterns, varied. She is messenger, mourner, saint, virgin, miracle, and witness, in addition to being a mother. She is found in devotional and artistic representations of all kinds. One of the myriads of representations popular in the Middle Ages and beyond is the Black Madonna. Michael Duricy defines Black Madonnas as "a type of Marian statue or painting of mainly medieval origin (12C–15C), of dark or black features whose exact origins are not always easy to determine, and most important, of particular prominence...due to the allegedly miraculous char-

47 Geoffroi de Charny, *A Knight's Own Book of Chivalry*, 95.

48 Geoffroi de Charny, *A Knight's Own Book of Chivalry*, 61.

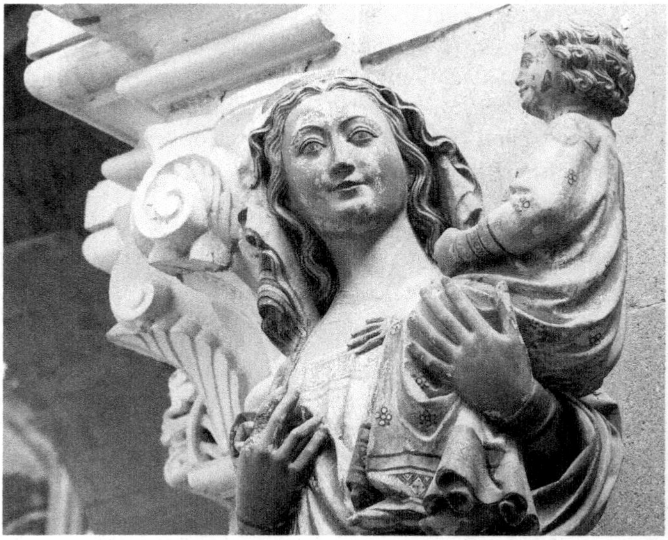

Figure 12. "Black Madonna," Magdeburg Cathedral, Germany, thirteenth century. Photograph by author.

acter of the image."[49] Hundreds of Black Madonnas have been catalogued across Europe in the Middle Ages.

The thirteenth-century Black Madonna at Magdeburg Cathedral in Germany is one example. Not as famous as others of its kind, it is nonetheless a striking representative of this genre, particularly given that at some point in the nineteenth century it underwent a "cleaning" that removed its darkened complexion (see Fig. 12).

Brief Overview of Black Madonna Tradition

Black Madonna statues and paintings each have their own unique stories and significance. Traditionally, the image of the Black Madonna is associated with verse 1:5 in Song of Songs. The exact translation of this verse has inspired much discussion. Some translate it "I am black, but beautiful," indicating an exceptionalism in this figure, a controversial idea she could be perceived as both black and beautiful. Others translate it to "and beautiful," which reduces the conflict between the two descriptors—beautiful in addition to being black, not in spite of being black. The image of the Black Madonna has survived beyond the Middle Ages. From that period until now, Black Madonna figures have appeared across the world.

---

49 Duricy, "Black Madonnas."

The Black Madonna Icon of Czestochowa, Poland

One of the most famous is the Black Madonna of Częstochowa, Poland. Like many of these Madonnas, its origins are shrouded in legend, preventing us from even being able to date the icon properly. Legend says it was perhaps created by St. Luke and discovered by St. Helena. Sources at the Jasna Góra Monastery indicate that the Madonna came from Constantinople in the fourteenth century.

When the Black Madonna was credited with saving Jasna Góra from a Swedish invasion in 1655, she was officially named the Queen and Protector of Poland.[50] Anna Hamling writes:

> Virgin Mary's suffering is the essence of the Polish soul, Polish culture, Polish Catholicism, Polish history and of all Polish mothers...*Our Lady of Częstochowa* has always stood as the epitome of perfect motherhood, loving and forgiving, protector of her children who shared her grief in losing her son to a violent death on the cross.[51]

There are several theories as to why Our Lady of Częstochowa is black-skinned, ranging from the connection to the Song of Songs verse to its Byzantine artistic attribution to the residual effects of a fire. Whatever the origin of her skin tone, the fact remains that she is venerated as both a religious and national icon, and she has been since the Middle Ages.

Her life at Jasna Góra was eventful. Supposedly, she was stolen from the monastery in 1430, but the thieves' horses miraculously refused to carry her very far. In frustration, the thieves then slashed the painting, leaving her with distinctive "scars" (and one of the thieves in death throes).

Black Madonnas in Black-Lives-Matter Imagery

The Black Madonna has more than simply survived beyond the Middle Ages. The representation has been adopted and redesigned for many purposes, none more poignant than the Black Lives Matter movement. Black Lives Matter artists have adapted the Black Madonna, particularly because of her position as a mother to a sacrificed son. One of the most well-known of these artists is Mark Dukes (or Doox) and his painting "Our Lady, Mother of Ferguson and All Those Killed by Gun Violence," or simply "Our Lady of Ferguson," which was created in 2016 in response to the Ferguson protests.

---

50 See Our Lady of Czestochowa Foundation, *The Glories of Czestochowa and Jasna Gora*; and Pasierb, *The Shrine of the Black Madonna.*

51 Hamling, "The Power of an Image."

Commissioned by Rev. Mark Francisco Bozzuti-Jones from Trinity Church in Manhattan, the piece depicts a Black Madonna with her hands raised, a reference to the "hands up, don't shoot" gesture, which is mirrored in the silhouette of Christ over her womb centred in the crosshairs of a gun. Mary is the grieving mother of a son wrongfully murdered in a state-sanctioned punishment, yet she is also a symbol of a dominant culture and religion in America. While the Black Madonna tradition was widespread in Europe during the Middle Ages and around the world since then, particularly through the African diaspora, it is not a tradition that is widely acknowledged in Western cultures. Centring the tradition demonstrates that Christianity has never been the province of one race, and doing so in the context of racially motivated police brutality lends religious empathy.

Theaster Gates' 2018 "Black Madonna" exhibition explores the historical image while pushing beyond it to see its metaphoric possibilities, particularly in expressing the Black American female experience.[52] Harmonia Rosales, in both her 2018 "New World Consciousness" and 2020 "Miss Education: Reclaiming Our Identity" exhibitions, used Marian imagery to question the erasure of the Black woman from the story of humanity and to return her to a centralized position.[53]

Mark Steven Greenfield's 2020 exhibition, simply titled "Black Madonna," depicts scenes of the Black experience turned into "revenge fantasies." Mary, often with her son, sits in the front, unaware that behind them, in one case, a Confederate statue is being torn down or a Ku Klux Klan member is being crucified. Greenfield, on choosing to use the Black Madonna, comments, "Fear of the 'other' often devolves into mindless hatred. Yet sometimes the path to empathy lies in the visualization of one's physical victimization—particularly when paired with a symbol that has come to be associated with universal love."[54] At first glance, this juxtaposition of violence and the image of Mary seems unsettling, incongruous even. Greenfield's "Black Madonna" exhibition highlights contrasting, yet interwoven aspects of Mary as mother. She is, on one hand, the grieving mother. On the other, she is, for many, an instantly recognizable symbol of both religious and maternal devotion and love. Her simultaneous occupation of these spaces invokes both sympathy and reverence.

52 "Theaster Gates."

53 "Harmonia Rosales | Miss Education." See also Manatakis, "Harmonia Rosales Repaints Classic Artworks."

54 Greenfield, *Black Madonna*.

Traumatic Grief in Mater Dolorosa Narratives

One of Mary's personas is as the universal *Mater Dolorosa*, or the Mother of Sorrows, also known as Our Lady of Compassion, Our Lady of Sorrows, and Our Lady of Seven Sorrows, among other names. Mary's seven sorrows focus either on the foreshadowing of her son's death—such as the prophecy of Simeon—or the actual act—the Crucifixion, the spearing of Christ's side, and the burial. The image of the grieving Mary became common after the mid-thirteenth century. A *Mater Dolorosa* altar in the monastery in Schönau, Germany is considered one of the first. The feast day of Our Lady of Sorrows was designated in 1423. One of the most iconic artworks to depict the sorrowing Mary, Michelangelo's *Pietà* in Saint Peter's Basilica, is a statue of Mary holding the dead body of Christ across her body, created in 1498–1499.

Literature and poetry from the Middle Ages on have tried to convey Mary's emotions. One such example is the fourteenth-century Middle English *Dispute Between Mary and the Cross*, which is a debate poem that follows Mary's complaints against the Cross for being the tool by which Christ is killed. A witness to the Crucifixion comes forward to describe Mary:

> His mild Mother stood next to Him,
> Looked upward, and she was woeful;
> A sword struck her through the breast;
> Out of the Cross the knife came though!
> This sight saw I myself—
> The sword of love through her did pierce—
> She fell swooning through that event (lines 330–36).[55]

This description emphasizes Mary's woe and how she fainted at the sight of her son's death, indicating how a mother feels the trauma visited upon the body of her son. Mary became a significant intercessory figure especially the Catholic tradition, the logic being: if you want the ear of the son, talk to his mother. The Magdeburg Black Madonna, as with many other Madonnas, holds an infant Christ in her arms, a visual representation of the relationship between mother and son.

55 Translation mine, with guidance from the glosses in the edition.

Mothers of the [Black Lives Matter] Movement

> "I was telling someone that I had this really bad pain in my stomach earlier, not knowing what had happened. But once I found out what happened, that was my son's pain that I was feeling. And I didn't even know."—RowVaughn Wells, mother of Tyre Nichols, who died after a police beating on January 7, 2023, in Memphis, Tennessee[56]

> "What was taken away from me was my only son that I can never get back. I'm scared and I feel like I'm about to fall apart."—Pauletta Johnson, mother of Amaree'ya Henderson, on the phone with her son when he was killed by police on April 26, 2023, in Kansas City, Kansas[57]

> "He gave my son the sentence he wanted him to have. He took him from me."—Laurie Littlejohn, mother of Jor'dell Richardson, who was killed in a police encounter on June 1, 2023, in Aurora, Colorado.[58]

> "I was never supposed to be planning a funeral for my 13-year-old baby."—Megan Reed, mother of Sinzae Reed, who was killed by neighbor on October 12, 2022, in Columbus, Ohio.[59]

The image of the grieving mother is more than an artistic metaphor. The "Mothers of the Movement" is a group comprised of the mothers of Black Americans who have been killed by the police, including Valerie Bell, mother of Sean Bell; Gwen Carr, mother of Eric Garner; Sybrina Fulton, mother of Trayvon Martin; and Geneva Reed-Veal, mother of Sandra Bland. These women have spoken out about the deaths of their children, working and advocating for law enforcement reform to prevent more deaths. In their public appearances, these mothers lay bare their grief in hopes of affecting change. The grief of these mothers—and the vicarious grief of mothers-to-be—echo the *Mater Dolorosa* tradition.

It is a description reminiscent of the grief experienced and projected by the "Mothers of the Movement." Valerie Bell, telling her story to the Oxford Union Society in London in 2017, said, "I knew I was going to give birth to my son on May 18, 1983, as a C-section. I didn't have any labor pains. The pains came upon my body on November 25th, 2006. Fifty shots by NYPD."[60]

---

56 Cowan, "Tyre Nichols' Death."

57 NewsOne Staff, "147 Black Men and Boys Killed by Police."

58 Gionet, "Protestors Follow Hearse to Remember Jor'dell Richardson."

59 Negussie, "Mother of Sinzae Reed."

60 OxfordUnion, "Black Lives Matter."

As a Minneapolis police officer knelt on his neck, George Floyd cried out for his mother. Larcenia Floyd passed away two years previously, but he invoked her with his dying words. In the protests that followed Floyd's death, an image surfaced of a young, pregnant Black woman carrying a sign in front of the US Capitol building that read, "We are not carrying for 9 months / Then struggling for 9 hours during labor / Just for you to kneel on their neck for 9 minutes!! Black Lives Matter." The protester, Thema, later commented, "The video of his death and hearing him cry out for his mother will forever be embedded in my head. I truly believe that when Mr. Floyd called out for his mother, all mothers were summoned, of all ages."[61]

The "Mothers of the Movement" are taking on this intercessor role for themselves, conveying their grief at the deaths of their children and telling their children's stories in order to communicate the effects of systemic racism and advocate against police violence.

Whitewashing as Trauma

In the introduction, I discussed the definition of "historical trauma" by Nathaniel Vincent Mohatt et al. and how the Substance Abuse and Mental Health Services Administration established that long-term and sustained loss of culture can have a deep and abiding effect on mental and physical health.[62] One method by which culture is erased is whitewashing, or the distortion of culture to exclude non-white people. Unfortunately, Black Madonnas have experienced this phenomenon almost literally. Arguably the most famous is that of the Black Madonna of Chartres Cathedral, a 1508 wooden replica of a thirteenth-century silver version, which controversially underwent a "restoration" in 2017 that removed the dark exterior, whitening the statue's complexion.

The Magdeburg Black Madonna was "cleaned" in the nineteenth century, also removing its dark complexion and whitening its skin. Whereas the Chartres Madonna is still at least visible for its notoriety, it is difficult even to locate the Magdeburg statue in the Cathedral because it bears little resemblance to Michael Duricy's definition. The guide brochure does point the statue out, making sure the visitor is made aware of its presence and its story, and it is difficult to fault the present Cathedral for actions taken centuries before. The Cathedral is also well-known for its Saint Maurice statue dating from around 1240, which is famous for its appropriately African features.

61 Koenig, "Pregnant Woman Hopes to Stand." See also MacIsaac, "This Pregnant Mother's Protest Sign."

62 Mohatt et al., "Historical Trauma as Public Narrative"; "Trauma and Violence."

The Magdeburg Black Madonna serves as a physical manifestation of both the traditionally traumatic grief a mother feels at the violent death of a child as well as the historical trauma of whitewashing and erasure.

STORIES: Grieving with the Eleanor Crosses

Twelve Monuments from Harby, Nottinghamshire, to London, between 1291–1295

In 1254, a thirteen-year-old Eleanor of Castile, daughter of Ferdinand III, was married to fifteen-year-old Edward, son of Henry III of England, who would become king upon his father's death in 1272. The marriage brokered a peaceful solution to the dispute over the land of Gascony, over which Edward was duke. Despite its arranged beginning for political reasons, the youth of the couple, and the deaths of several infant children, they apparently developed a deep love and affection for each other. Sources indicate that they were rarely separated, even travelling together to Acre in the Crusades. Indeed, there is a (perhaps legendary) story of how, when Edward was the victim of an assassination attempt in Acre, Eleanor saved him by sucking the poison out of a knife wound.

In 1290, the now-Queen Eleanor and Edward I began a tour of her holdings in England on the way to Scotland. There were already indications that she was ill, possibly weakened from malaria or from complications after the birth of her last child (the last of at least sixteen births), and the travelling slowed down and became more difficult. Finally, in Harby, Nottinghamshire, on November 28, 1290, Eleanor of Castile died with her husband by her bedside.[63]

Eleanor's reputation during her life seems to have been quite mixed, to the point that Abigail S. Armstrong calls her the "consort of contradictions." As a Spaniard, she faced some suspicion in England, and the extensive land granted to her was a source of controversy, particularly because it was tied to her assumption of Jewish debts and to the Jewish expulsion in 1275. On the other hand, she was considered a pious woman, a patron of the arts, a skilled diplomat, and a dedicated wife and mother.[64]

Edward's grief was poignantly apparent. He wrote to the Abbot of Cluny, describing her as "our most serene consort," "who while living we loved dearly, and in death we do not cease to love."[65] After her death, Eleanor's body—with the exception of some of her organs that were buried at

---

63 For biographical information, see Cockerill, *Eleanor of Castile.*

64 See Armstrong, "Eleanor of Castile."

65 Armstrong, "Eleanor of Castile," 254.

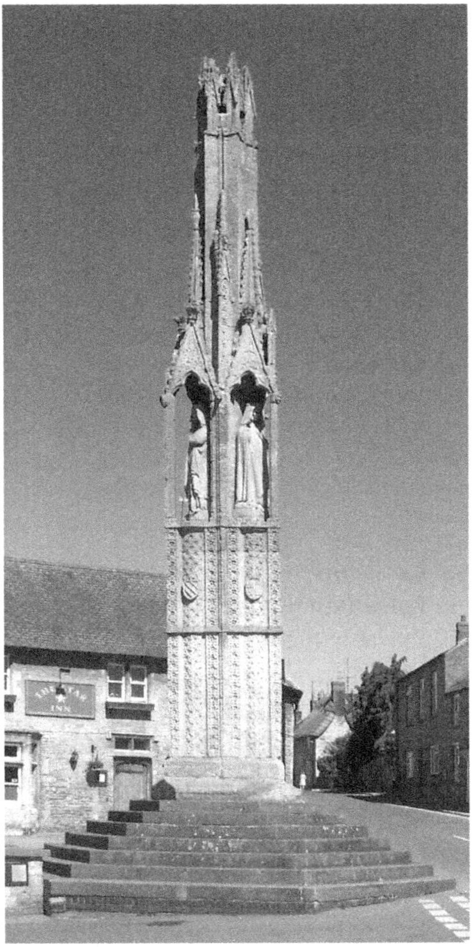

Figure 13. Eleanor cross, Geddington, Northamptonshire, England. Photograph by Lofty. CC BY 2.5.

Lincoln Cathedral—was carried in a funeral procession from Harby to Westminster Abbey, stopping several times along the way. At each of those twelve stops, Edward had a monument erected to memorialize his wife: "The King undertook a massive programme of funerary monuments and commemoration, with effigies at the three different sites of her burial and twelve crosses, one at each of the locations her body lay overnight on the journey back to London."[66] These monuments, which came to be known as the Eleanor crosses, are tall, with royal arms and statues of Eleanor (see the Geddington cross in Fig. 13). They might also at one time have had crosses on top, but more likely the "crosses" refer to their positioning at crossroads. Eleanor is represented with a bowed head and a sceptre in her right hand, perhaps drawing on "Marian imagery to present Eleanor as submissive and graceful."[67] Only three of these monuments have survived intact, having suffered from the iconoclasm of the Reformation and the English Civil War.[68]

While the construction and the design of the crosses undeniably had political purposes, our focus is on their representation of grief and how monuments can play a role in the healing of trauma, for, as the political meaning lost its prominence with time, the emotional gained legendary status: "Memorials serve an important remembering function not because they restore living memory, but because they symbolically articulate and engage

66 Armstrong, "Eleanor of Castile," 253.

67 Davies, *Visions and Ruins*, 74.

68 See the Introduction for more on iconoclasm.

with the fragility and temporality of living memory's mortality."[69] Indeed, even Edward's potential aim to rehabilitate his wife's reputation with the monuments is an act of diplomacy, but it is also an act of grieving remembrance. We can argue that he achieved both, as Eleanor's lasting legacy seems to be more one of a memorialized wife than a controversial ruler. Joshua Davies examines this aspect of the Eleanor crosses:

> Famously, their origins apparently begin with the trauma of an early death and the grief of Edward I but...the crosses were deeply political and more committed to reimagining than remembering the past. They fashioned an idealised image of Eleanor that stands distinct from the historical record but defined cultural memories of her. Over time, however, what were once memorials to an individual woman came to signify a more general sense of loss, melancholy and nostalgia that spoke to particular times, places and experiences.[70]

This latter sense of general loss is attested by the influence the crosses had on the designer of the Albert Memorial in Kensington Gardens, which was built in 1872 at the commission of Queen Victoria in memory of the queen's Royal Consort, Prince Albert—the private grief of royalty again commemorated in public spaces. Brady Wagoner and Ignacio Brescó de Luna comment on the death of public figures, stating that "people feel the need to meet in public spaces and express themselves with other members of the community."[71] These monuments are symbols of both the traumatic grief of a devoted husband as well as the performed grief of a nation, and they have become a more universal symbol of loss.

Contexts: Addressing Stigma

Stigma has followed disability through the centuries and has complicated its representations. The medieval representations of disability are no different. There are positive representations, with various forms of impairment associated with holiness—particularly in hagiography—as well as the inclusion of people with disabilities in all kinds of art forms and non-exclusionary burial practices. On the other hand, there are negative views as well. The story of the prostitute in the *Book of the Foundation of St. Bartholomew's Church* presents disability as a consequence of sinful behaviour. The young

---

69 Gibson, "Death and Grief in the Landscape," 150.

70 Davies, *Visions and Ruins*, 68.

71 Wagoner and de Luna, "Collective Grief," 197.

woman is punished with both mental and physical disabilities as a result of her choices to engage in deviant sexual behaviour. The fourteenth-century Middle English sermon that equates leprosy with sin has a similar approach, using the outward manifestations of the disease as a metaphor for inward evil.

Not all representations are so clear. The role of disability in the Aztec empire and in Moctezuma's court in particular is complicated, revealing not only apparent locations that put people with disability on display but also the social positions that place them in proximity to power.[72] In *African Myths of Origin*, there is a Yoruban myth that describes the creation of humans by the orishas (or deities) Obatala and Olorun, and also presents a blend of positive and negative connotations of disability.[73] During this creation, Olorun forms some humans out of clay while intoxicated, which is the myth's explanation for some physical disabilities:

> Obatala began to make figures of clay. Olorun breathed life into them. They became people whom Obatala placed in his new land. Other orisha came down from heaven to join him in the new land. Olorun created the sun and moon to give them light. The sun made Obatala thirsty, and he drank the fermented sap of the palm tree. The palm wine made him drunk, and some of the human figures he made at that time were deformed or incomplete. He fell asleep after a while; when he woke he saw that he had done, and regretted having brought misshapen people into the world. He swore never to drink palm wine again, and he became the protector of the children of his drunkenness.[74]

In this story, we can see an approach to categorizing people with disabilities as an inadvertent part of creation. Yet, at the same time, their creation is still a natural (as opposed to unnatural, or against nature) consequence of a deity becoming thirsty under a newly-created sun and drinking fermented sap. There is a reference to "regret" for this creation, although this translation would need to be investigated more closely. In the end, the orisha designates himself as the protector of people with disabilities, indicating that they are in some ways divine and thus respected.

---

72 See Bearden, *Monstrous Kinds*, 109–41.

73 See Chapter 2's "Contexts: The Language of Disability" for discussion of the translation issues of this text.

74 *African Myths of Origin*, ed. Belcher, 311.

Faking Disability

One representation that reinforces some of the negativity has nothing to do with the people with disabilities themselves, but rather those who fake disability in order to swindle or for some other personal gain. This fear seems to permeate how people perceive people with actual disabilities, because there is a sense of distrust mixed with a concern not to be swindled.

In the fourteenth-century *Decameron* by Italian author Giovanni Boccaccio, one of the stories centres on three men who arrive in Treviso not long after the death of Saint Arrigo (2.1). Curious to see the saint's body, they are frustrated by the guards placed around him and the throngs of people. One of them, Martellino, devises a plan:

> I will counterfeit a paralytic, and thou wilt support me on one side and Stecchi on the other, as if I were not able to go alone, and so you will enter the church, making it appear as if you were leading me up to the body of the saint that he may heal me, and all that see will make way and give us free passage.[75]

A professional actor skilled in impersonation, "Martellino distorted his hands, his fingers, his arms, his legs, and also his mouth and eyes and his entire face in a manner horrible to contemplate; so that no stranger that saw him could have doubted that he was impotent and paralysed in every part of his body." After his friends lead him to the saint's body in the church, the actor then pretends to be miraculously healed: "being a very practised performer, he stretched, first, one of his fingers, next a hand, afterwards an arm, and so forth, making as if he gradually recovered the use of all his natural powers." Although giving a very adept performance that was at first hailed with astonishment, Martellino is revealed by someone who happens to know him, and the people "dragged him down from where he stood, seized him by the hair, tore the clothes from his back, and fell to beating and kicking him." He is taken by the guards and, having been brought before a legal authority, is on the verge of being hanged when he is saved by an acquaintance. The violent reaction of the people in the church to Martellino's deception is telling, as it indicates, first, a level of acceptance of his supposed condition, followed by extreme disgust at someone who would exploit it, not to mention who was so good at it that he was able initially to fool them.

---

75 Boccaccio, *The Decameron*, trans. Rigg. *The Decameron* is divided into a series of volumes described as "days," which each contain a series "novels," or books. This scene comes from the first "novel" of the second "day," and thus is represented as (2.1).

In *Dissembling Disability in Early Modern English Drama*, Lindsey Row-Heyveld notes a continued, if not increased, concern with falsifying disability in the Early Modern period. That people with disabilities suffer as a result of a few who would exploit their circumstances is certainly unfair.

Consequences of Stigma

Unfortunately, one of the consequences of stigma is violence enacted against people with disabilities, which has been a part of their story for a long time, and the Middle Ages is no different. The "Mad" Henry of the Fordwich stained glass at Canterbury Cathedral depicts the beating of a man in the midst of a mental health episode. Other miracles in the *Book of the Foundation of St. Bartholomew's Church* describe "mad" individuals being bound. These are just a few examples that speak to a wider problem of abuse against vulnerable individuals—a problem that continues in the modern day.

Humour Reinforcing Stigma

In *Stumbling Blocks Before the Blind: Medieval Constructions of a Disability*, Edward Wheatley dedicates an entire chapter to the "comic embodiment of blindness." He details examples of texts with "the express purpose of humiliating blind characters or placing them in degrading situations for comic ends."[76] He points out "ballads, fabliaux, farces, and a romance," finding that "the deployment of stereotypes about blind people and related plot devices transcends genre."[77] These stereotypes are not confined only to Blind characters; other disabilities also, at times, receive similar treatment.

Humour is not limited to the written word but can be found even in something that appears as innocuous as children's games, such as Blind Man's Bluff (see Fig. 14). Represented in a fourteenth-century French Breviary (London, British Library, Yates Thompson MS 8, fol. 92), it is on the surface simply a game with someone blindfolded in the middle who tries to tag the other players; however, like many historical children's games, it has sinister overtones. At times, this game has been played with the others tagging or even hitting the player in the middle, as they flail around attempting to find them. The player in the middle is metaphorically blind, and these actions mock that condition, perhaps even performing violence on such individuals.

---

76 Wheatley, *Stumbling Blocks Before the Blind*, 90.

77 Wheatley, *Stumbling Blocks Before the Blind*, 91.

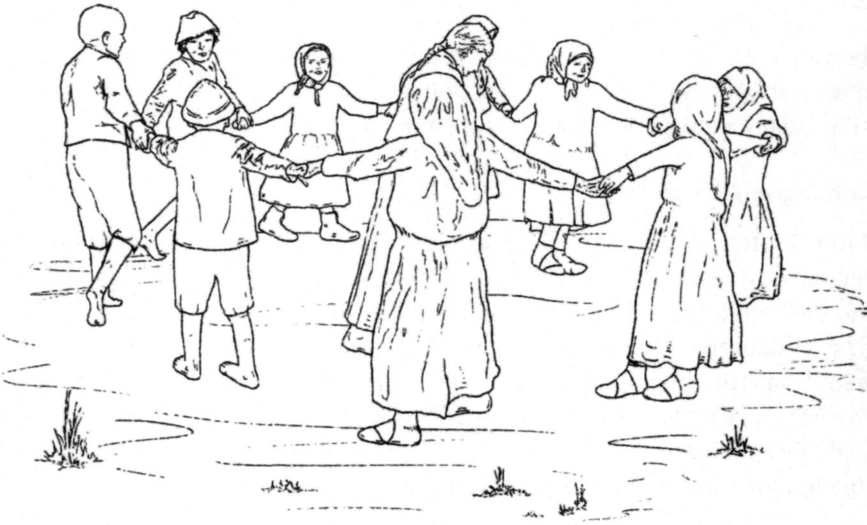

Figure 14. A game of Blind Man's Bluff.
Illustration by Dayanna Knight. Reproduced with permission.

The best way to counter the stigma associated with disability is to make it visible and to make sure it is represented in respectful and accurate ways in every aspect of culture. As this exhibition has hopefully proven, disability has a long heritage with complex and impactful stories. These stories need to be told.

Epilogue

THE SIGNIFICANCE OF MEDIEVAL DISABILITY HERITAGE

ACCORDING TO THE Centers of Disease Control and Prevention, more than 1 in 4 adults in the United States has some type of disability.[1] According to the World Health Organization, approximately 1.3 billion people experience significant disability, which is 16% of the world's population, or 1 in 6.[2] Given these statistics, it is possible that everyone either has or knows someone who has a disability. It is also an identity that anyone may enter into at any time in their lives, whether through disease, accident, acts of violence, or age.

These facts increase the need for engaging with disability heritage. Disability did not appear in the modern era; it has always existed. Cultural heritage is the manifestation of common human experiences, and, by drawing parallels between medieval and modern disabilities, we can emphasize those connections through the shared need for preservation and the study of the premodern. In addition to continuing to discover and uncover new artifacts—such as through archaeological excavations—some of the work that needs to be done is a matter of (re)interpretation, of looking at existing heritage through the lens of disability, such as the discussions of the Black Madonna or the Cōātlīcue statue in this exhibition.

Thinking about the body is particularly important to disability studies. Much of what we can learn about physical disabilities is written on our bodies, and examining human anatomy reveals a wealth of information. This information, however, is tied to respecting the dignity of those bodies, both living and diseased. Respect for human remains translates to respect for human beings more generally, which can counter stigma and improve the well-being of those experiencing disability.

Disability is also associated with many artifacts of material culture, as accommodating a disability may require physical technology, such as hand-trestles, walking sticks, or prosthetics. In the premodern world, these accommodations were the product of human ingenuity without the benefit of modern technologies to ease the way. The daily life of those with disabilities includes a variety of people, communities of care, caregivers, and even

1 Centers of Disease Control and Prevention, "Disability Impacts All of Us."

2 World Health Organization, "Disability."

DOI: 10.17302/asgs32688 © Arc Humanities Press

animals, such as guide dogs. These communities—whether in hospitals or less institutionalized forms—have their own heritage, and they leave their own traces and stories. To decipher these traces requires interdisciplinary study of a variety of sources and interaction with a number of languages, which may be filtered through translators and interpreters who may or may not have agendas or prejudices of their own.

Certain disabilities, such as mental or cognitive ones, may not leave as much tangible evidence as physical ones. These do not always require accommodation through technologies and may not leave a mark on our bodies. Nonetheless, uncovering these stories is necessary to understanding the historical experiences of all people.

Erasing or ignoring people with disabilities in our quest to understand human nature denies the parts of us that respond to vulnerabilities, our own or someone else's. It excises from the record a substantial portion of the population, both past and present. The positive experiences of those with differences illuminate what we are capable of, what we can invent, and what we can do as communities. Even in studying moments when the treatment of people with disabilities is negative, and thus revealing the cruelty of which we are capable, we learn. We learn how to be better and do better in our present world.

Medieval disability cultural heritage is our passport, a way to visit a different time, perhaps a different geography, and meet people with stories that educate and move us.

BIBLIOGRAPHY

Primary Sources

African Myths of Origin. Selected and retold by Stephen Belcher. Penguin, 2005.

Arano, Luisa Cogliati. *The Medieval Health Handbook: Tacuinum sanitatis*. Translated by Oscar Ratti and Adele Westbrook. Braziller, 1976.

Basilakes, Nikephoros. "Encomium." In *The Rhetorical Exercises of Nikephoros Basilakes*, edited and translated by Jeffrey Beneker and Craig A. Gibson, 129–43. Harvard University Press, 2016.

Benedict of Peterborough. *The Passion and Miracles of St. Thomas Becket by Benedict of Peterborough*. Translated by Rachel Koopmans. Studies in the History of Medieval Religion. Boydell & Brewer, 2025.

Boccaccio, Giovanni. *The Decameron*. Translated by J. M. Rigg. Project Gutenberg, 2003. https://gutenberg.org/cache/epub/3726/pg3726.html.

Book of the Foundation of St. Bartholomew's Church. Edited by Humphrey H. King and William Barnard. Rahere's Garden, 2005. https://www.raheresgarden.org/Book-of-the-Foundation.pdf.

British Museum. "Cartonnage (Prosthetic Toe)." https://www.britishmuseum.org/collection/object/Y_EA29996.

Chaucer, Geoffrey. *The Canterbury Tales and Other Works*. Librarius, 1997. http://www.librarius.com/.

Conrad, David C., ed. and trans. *Sunjata: A West African Epic of the Mande Peoples*. Narrated by Djanka Tassey Condé. Hackett, 2004.

"The Dispute Between Mary and the Cross." In *Moral Love Songs and Laments*, edited by Susanna Greer Fein. Middle English Texts Series. TEAMS, Medieval Institute, 1998.

Edward of Norwich. *The Master of Game: The Oldest English Book on Hunting*. Edited by F. Baillie-Grohman and William A. Baillie-Grohman. Project Gutenberg, 2024. https://www.gutenberg.org/files/43452/43452-h/43452-h.htm.

"Egils Saga." *wikisaga*, last edited October 26, 2011. https://wikisaga.hi.is/index.php?title=Category:Egils_saga._Efnisyfirlit.

Egyptian Museum. "Prosthetic Toe of Tabaket en Mut." https://egypt-museum.com/prosthetic-toe-of-tabaket-en-mut/.

Froissart, Jean. "Jean Froissart: On the Hundred Years War (1337–1453)." *Medieval Sourcebook*. Fordham University Press, 1996. https://sourcebooks.web.fordham.edu/source/froissart1.asp.

Geoffroi de Charny. *A Knight's Own Book of Chivalry*. Translated by Elspeth Kennedy. University of Pennsylvania Press, 2005.

Greenfield, Mark Steven. *Black Madonna*. William Turner Gallery. issuu, 2020. https://issuu.com/turnergallery/docs/mark_steven_greenfield.

Hanham, Alison. *Richard III and His Early Historians, 1483–1535*. Clarendon, 1975.

DOI: 10.17302/asgs32689 © Arc Humanities Press

"Harmonia Rosales | Miss Education: Reclaiming Our Identity," Museum of Contemporary African Diasporan Arts. https://mocada.org/harmonia-rosales-miss-education-reclaiming-our-identity/.

Horstmann, Carl. "Prosalegenden: Die Legenden des MS Douce 114." *Anglia* 8 (1885): 134–84.

The Iroquois Book of Rites. Edited by Horatio Hale. Brinton's Library of Aboriginal American Literature. Project Gutenberg, 2012. https://www.gutenberg.org/cache/epub/8567/pg8567-images.html.

Japanese Tales from Times Past: Stories of Fantasy and Folklore from the Konjaku Monogatari Shu. Translated by Naoshi Koriyama and Bruce Allen. Tuttle, 2015.

Lucid, Nancy. "Medicinal Plant List for the St. Clare Garden." *Santa Clara University*, 2005. https://www-archive.scu.edu/media/offices/st-clare-garden/pdfs/medicinal_rev.pdf.

Lucid, Nancy. "St. Clare Garden." *Santa Clara University.* https://www.scu.edu/stclaregarden/.

Merchant Culture in Fourteenth-Century Venice: The Zibaldone da Canal. Edited and translated by John Dotson. Medieval and Renaissance Texts and Studies, 1994.

Middle English Legends of Women Saints. Edited by Sherry L. Reames. Medieval Institute, 2003. http://d.lib.rochester.edu/teams/publication/reames-middle-english-legends-of-women-saints.

Niane, D. T. *Sundiata: An Epic of Old Mali.* Translated by G. D. Pickett. Longman, 1965.

Orlemanski, Julie. "Leprosy." *Medieval Disability Glossary.* https://medievaldisabilityglossary.hcommons.org/leprosy/.

Ovid. *Metamorphoses.* Translated by Samuel Garth, John Dryden, et al. *Internet Classics Archive.* https://classics.mit.edu/Ovid/metam.html.

Perkins School for the Blind. "Blind in Art Collection." https://www.perkins.org/finding-aid/blind-in-art/.

Perkins School for the Blind. "Spring on the Yellow River, 13th-Century Chinese Scroll with Seeing Eye Dog." *Digital Commonwealth.* https://www.digitalcommonwealth.org/search/commonwealth:vx022057g.

Saints' Lives in Middle English Collections. Edited by E. Gordon Whatley, Anne B. Thompson, and Robert K. Upchurch. Medieval Institute, 2004. https://d.lib.rochester.edu/teams/publication/whatley-saints-lives-in-middle-english-collections.

Smithsonian Archives of American Art. "Monuments Men Series." https://www.aaa.si.edu/resources/excerpts-from-the-archives-oral-history-interviews.

Thaut, Michael H. "Music as Therapy in Early History." *Progress in Brain Research*, 217 (2015): 143–58.

"Theaster Gates: Black Madonna." *Kunstmuseum Basel.* https://kunstmuseumbasel.ch/en/exhibitions/2018/gates, accessed December 25, 2025.

Tracy, Kisha G., and Alicia Protze. "Life of Mary of Oegines (Oignies) (ca. 15th c.)." In *Medieval Disability Sourcebook: Western Europe*, edited by Cameron Hunt McNabb, 220–30. punctum, 2020.

"Translation of Alfred's Prose Preface to Pastoral Care." Bucknell University. https://www.departments.bucknell.edu/english/courses/engl440/pastoral/translation.shtml.

Tree+. "The Peacemaker & the Tadadaho." Posted September 17, 2015, YouTube, 10 min. https://youtu.be/9iVziGHPhVw?si=KloJWeO5SY2RVAbm.

Yale Library. "Arthurian Romances." https://collections.library.yale.edu/catalog/2004282.

Secondary Works

Agnew, Hugh L. *The Czechs and the Lands of the Bohemian Crown*. Hoover, 2004.

Alberti, Samuel J. M. M. "Objects and the Museum." *Isis* 96, no. 4 (2005): 559–71.

American Association of Neurological Surgeons. "Scoliosis." April 30, 2024. https://www.aans.org/patients/conditions-treatments/scoliosis/.

American Bookbinders Museum. "The Cottonian Library Fire." February 29, 2016. https://bookbindersmuseum.org/cottonian-library-fire/.

Anderson, T., and T. Glyn Thomas. "A Possible Case of Arthrogryposis Multiplex from Medieval Canterbury." *International Journal of Osteoarchaeology* 7 (1997): 181–85.

Angenendt, Arnold. "Relics and Their Veneration." In *Treasures of Heaven: Saints, Relics, and Devotion in Medieval Europe*, edited by Martina Bagnoli et al., 19–28. Cleveland Museum of Art, 2010.

Appleby, Jo, et al. "The Scoliosis of Richard III, Last Plantagenet King of England: Diagnosis and Clinical Significance." *The Lancet* 383, no. 9932 (2014): 1944.

Armstrong, Abigail S. "Eleanor of Castile: A Consort of Contradictions." In *Norman to Early Plantagenet Consorts: Queenship and Power*, edited by Aidan Norrie et al., 237–55. Palgrave Macmillan, 2023.

Ashmore, Kevin, et al. "ArtiFacts: Gottfried 'Götz' von Berlichingen-The 'Iron Hand' of the Renaissance." *Clin Orthop Relat Res* 477, no. 9 (2019): 2002–4.

Barakat, Robert A. "Cistercian Sign Language." In *Monastic Sign Languages*, edited by Jean Umiker-Sebeok, 67–323. De Gruyter, 1987.

Barakat, Robert A. "On Ambiguity in the Cistercian Sign Language." *Sign Language Studies*, no. 8 (1975): 275–89.

Barts Health Archives. "Research Guide: Medieval Records of St Bartholomew's Hospital." *Barts Health NHS Trust* 3 (2025). https://www.calmview.co.uk/BartsHealth/CalmView/Medieval%20records%20v0.3.pdf.

Bearden, Elizabeth B. *Monstrous Kinds: Body, Space, and Narrative in Renaissance Representations of Disability*. University of Michigan Press, 2019.

Bednarska, Dominika. "Rethinking Access: Why Technology Isn't the Only Answer." In *The Culture of Efficiency: Technology in Everyday Life*, edited by Sharon Kleinman, 158–69. Lang, 2009.

Belcastro, Maria Giovanna, and Valentina Mariotti. "The Place of Human Remains in the Frame of Cultural Heritage: The Restitution of Medieval Skeletons from a Jewish Cemetery." *Journal of Cultural Heritage* 49 (2021): 229–38.

Bell, Clive. "Art." In *Historical and Philosophical Issues in the Conservation of Cultural Heritage*, edited by Nicholas Stanley-Price, M. Kirby Talley, Jr., and Alessandra Melucco Vaccaro, 47–55. Getty, 1996.

Berger, John. *Ways of Seeing*. Penguin, 1972.

Binder, Michaela, et al. "Prosthetics in Antiquity—An Early Medieval Wearer of a Foot Prosthesis (6th Century AD) from Hemmaberg/Austria." *International Journal of Paleopathology* 12 (2016): 29–40.

Boehm, Barbara Drake. "Relics and Reliquaries in Medieval Christianity." *The Met Timeline of Art History*, October 1, 2001, revised April 1, 2011. https://www.metmuseum.org/essays/relics-and-reliquaries-in-medieval-christianity.

Bortolot, Alexander Ives. "Women Leaders in African History: Idia, First Queen Mother of Benin." *Heilbrunn Timeline of Art History*, The Metropolitan Museum of Art, 2003. https://www.metmuseum.org/toah/hd/pwmn_3/hd_pwmn_3.htm.

Bouttiaux, Anne-Marie, and Marc Ghysels. "Scrofulous Sogolon—Scanning the Sunjata Epic." *Tribal Art* 75 (2015): 88–123.

Brenner, Elma. *Leprosy and Charity in Medieval Rouen*. Boydell & Brewer, 2015.

Brentari, Diane. *Sign Languages: A Cambridge Language Survey*. Cambridge University Press, 2010.

Broerken, Egbert. "Take a Walk Through the Streets on Your Fingertips." https://egbert-broerken.com/41557.html.

Brubaker, Leslie. *Inventing Byzantine Iconoclasm*. Bristol, 2012.

Bruce, Scott G. *Silence and Sign Language in Medieval Monasticism: The Cluniac Tradition c. 900–1200*. Cambridge University Press, 2007.

Bryant, Richard. "Post-Traumatic Stress Disorder VS Traumatic Brain Injury." *Dialogues in Clinical Neuroscience* 13, no. 3 (2011): 251–62.

Bryner, Jeanna. "Painful Treatment Possible for King Richard III's Scoliosis." *NBC News*, April 19, 2013. https://www.nbcnews.com/sciencemain/painful-treatment-possible-king-richard-iiis-scoliosis-1b9520980.

Buck, Christopher. "Deganawida, the Peacemaker." In *American Writers, Supplement XXVI*, edited by Jay Parini, 81–100. Scribner, 2015.

Burgess, W. G. "Time's Teeth: Narratives of Preservation in the Eighteenth-Century Cotton Library." *Notes and Records of the Royal Society of London* 76, no. 2 (2022): 303–15.

Buterin, Toni, Amir Muzur, and Bojan Glažar. "Saints and 'Possession': A Case Review Bordering Ethnopsychiatry and Cultural Diversity." *Journal of Religion and Health* 60 (2021): 1116–24.

Byock, Jesse. "Egil's Bones." *Scientific American* 272, no. 1 (1995): 82–87.

Byock, Jesse. "The Skull and Bones in Egils Saga: A Viking, A Grave, and Paget's Disease." *Viator* 24 (1993): 23–50.

California Missions Foundation. "History of Mission Santa Clara de Asís." https://californiamissionsfoundation.org/mission-santa-clara/.

Callahan, Christopher. "Music in Medieval Medical Practice: Speculations and Certainties." *College Music Symposium* 40 (2000): 151–64.

Canterbury Historical and Archaeological Society. "Miracle Windows North Aisle." June 2025. https://www.canterbury-archaeology.org.uk/miracle-windows-north-aisle.

Castelow, Ellen. "The Battle of Towton." *HistoricUK*. https://www.historic-uk.com/HistoryMagazine/DestinationsUK/The-Battle-of-Towton/.

Caucasus Heritage Watch, "Silent Erasure: A Satellite Investigation of the Destruction of Armenian Cultural Heritage in Nakhchivan, Azerbaijan." *StoryMaps*, October 2, 2024. https://storymaps.arcgis.com/stories/48703f664f2f467b8f4f42008d8c75da.

Centers of Disease Control and Prevention. "Disability Impacts All of Us." April 14, 2025. https://www.cdc.gov/disability-and-health/articles-documents/disability-impacts-all-of-us-infographic.html.

Centers for Disease Control and Prevention. "Living with Down Syndrome." November 22, 2024. https://www.cdc.gov/birth-defects/living-with-down-syndrome/?CDC_AAref_Val=https://www.cdc.gov/ncbddd/birthdefects/downsyndrome/data.html.

Christoph, Henning. "The Secret of the Putchu Guinadji." *Soul of Africa Museum,* 2013. https://www.soul-of-africa.com/en/exhibitions/healing.html?file=files/content/ausstellungen/heilung_und_schutz/THE%20SECRET%20OF%20THE%20PUTCHU%20GUINADJI.pdf.

Clanchy, M. T. "'Tenacious Letters': Archives and Memory in the Middle Ages." *Archivaria* no. 11 (1980–1981): 115–25.

Cleall, Esme. "Disability and Postcolonialism." *Postcolonial Studies* 27, no. 1 (2024): 1–16.

Cockerill, Sara. *Eleanor of Castile: The Shadow Queen.* Amberley, 2014.

Columbia University Graduate School of Architecture, Planning and Preservation. "The Preservation of Disability." https://www.arch.columbia.edu/events/1953-the-preservation-of-disability.

"Convention for the Safeguarding of the Intangible Cultural Heritage." *United Nations Educational, Scientific and Cultural Organization*, October 17, 2003. https://ich.unesco.org/en/convention.

Cook, Lindsay. "Leaving a Trace." *Vassar*, November 16, 2023. https://www.vassar.edu/news/leaving-a-trace.

Council for British Archaeology. "Overlooked but on Display: Disability and Human Remains in Museums." *YouTube*, August 30, 2022. https://youtu.be/3pZFuWjmm3k?si=bwWjOGaAAsZ4_ONj, accessed 6 July 2026.

Cowan, Lee. "Tyre Nichols' Death, and a Mother's Pain." *CBS News*, January 29, 2023. https://www.cbsnews.com/news/tyre-nichols-death-and-a-mothers-pain/.

Crane, Susan. *Animal Encounters: Contacts and Concepts in Medieval Britain.* University of Pennsylvania Press, 2012.

Cultural Heritage Preservation: The Past, the Present and the Future. Edited by Tomas Nilson and Kristina Thorell. Halmstad University, 2018. https://www.diva-portal.org/smash/get/diva2:1224014/FULLTEXT01.pdf.

Daley, Jason. "This 3,000-Year-Old Wooden Toe Shows Early Artistry of Prosthetics." *The Smithsonian Magazine*, June 21, 2017. https://www.smithsonianmag.com/smart-news/study-reveals-secrets-ancient-cairo-toe-180963783/.

Davies, Joshua. *Visions and Ruins: Cultural Memory and the Untimely Middle Ages.* Manchester University Press, 2018.

Dean and Chapter of Canterbury Cathedral. "Stained Glass in Canterbury Cathedral." *Canterbury Cathedral.* https://learning.canterbury-cathedral.org/how-did-they-build-that/stained-glass/.

Decision Makers of Luxembourg. "John the Blind (King of Bohemia): The Legend of a Knight." *360Crossmedia*, 2025. https://www.decisionmakersluxembourg.com/johntheblind.

De León, Ann. "Coatlicue or How to Write the Dismembered Body." *MLN* 125, no. 2 (2010): 259–86.

de Vos, Connie, and Ulrike Zeshan. "Introduction: Demographic, Sociocultural, and Linguistic Variation across Rural Signing Communities." In *Sign Languages in Village Communities: Anthropological and Linguistic Insights*, edited by Ulrike Zeshan and Connie de Vos, 2–24. De Gruyter, 2012.

de Witte, Bruno. "Language as Cultural Heritage." In *The Oxford Handbook of International Cultural Heritage Law*, edited by Francesco Francioni and Ana Filipa Vrdoljak, 371–78. Oxford University Press, 2020.

Diebold, William. "The Nazi Middle Ages." In *Whose Middle Ages? Teachable Moments for an Ill-Used Past*, edited by Andrew Albin et al., 104–15. Fordham University Press, 2019.

Displaced Heritage: Responses to Disaster, Trauma, and Loss. Edited by Ian Convery, Gerard Corsane, and Peter Davis. Boydell & Brewer, 2014.

Duricy, Michael. "Black Madonnas: Origin, History, Controversy." *All About Mary*, University of Dayton. https://udayton.edu/imri/mary/b/black-madonnas-origin-history-controversy.php.

Dwyer, Philip. "Destroying the Past: A History of Iconoclasm." *Philip Dwyer*, 2024. https://www.philip-dwyer.com/current-projects/destroying-the-past%3A-a-history-of-iconoclasm.

el Damaty, Sarah, Simon Hazubski, and Andreas Otte. "ArtiFacts: Creating a 3-D CAD Reconstruction of the Historical Roman Capua Leg." *Clinical Orthopaedics and Related Research* 479, no. 9 (2021): 1911–13.

Farrar, Tarikhu. "The Queenmother, Matriarchy, and the Question of Female Political Authority in Precolonial West African Monarchy." *Journal of Black Studies* 27, no. 5 (1997): 579–97.

Favor, Lesli J. *The Iroquois Constitution: A Primary Source Investigation of the Law of the Iroquois*. Rosen, 2003.

Fiorato, Veronica. "The Context of the Discovery." In *Blood Red Roses: The archaeology of a mass grave from the Battle of Towton AD 1461*, edited by Veronica Fiorato, Anthea Boylston, and Christopher Knüsel, 1–14. Oxbow, 2007.

Fly, Erin Suzanne. "Multicultural Music Therapy: Exploring the Approaches to, and Changes in, Music within the Native American Communities." Master's thesis, University of Missouri-Kansas City, 2010.

Foys, Martin. "Medieval Manuscripts: Media Archaeology and the Digital Incunable." In *The Medieval Manuscript Book: Cultural Approaches*, edited by M. Van Dussen and M. Johnston, 119–39. Cambridge University Press, 2015.

Frigerio, Alberto. "Heritage Under Attack: A Critical Analysis of the Reasons Behind the Destruction of Cultural Property in the Event of Armed Conflict." *Aedon* 2 (2014). http://www.aedon.mulino.it/archivio/2014/2/frigerio.htm.

Garland-Thomson, Rosemarie. *Staring: How We Look*. Oxford University Press, 2009.

Gibson, Margaret. "Death and Grief in the Landscape: Private Memorials in Public Space." *Cultural Studies Review* 17, no. 1 (2011): 146–61.

Gionet, Alan. "Protestors Follow Hearse to Remember Jor'dell Richardson Who Died after Being Shot by Aurora Police." *CBS News*, June 17, 2023. https://www.cbsnews.com/colorado/news/protestors-follow-hearse-remember-jordell-richardson-killed-aurora-police/.

Gordon, Eleanora C. "Arthrogryposis Multiplex Congenita, AD 1156." *Developmental Medicine & Child Neurology* 38, no. 1 (1996): 80–83.

Hagen, K. M. H. *Miraculous Crosses and Crucifixes in Late Medieval and Early Modern Norway*. Palgrave Macmillan, 2024.

Hamilton, Bernard. *The Leper King and His Heirs: Baldwin IV and the Crusader Kingdom of Jerusalem*. Cambridge University Press, 2000.

Hamling, Anna. "The Power of an Image: The Black Madonna of Czestochowa," *Think International Academic Forum*, March 30, 2017. https://think.iafor.org/the-power-of-an-image-the-black-madonna-of-czestochowa/.

Haneca, Kristof, and Marjan Buyle. "The Reliquary of Saint Dymphna: Dating Wood and Bones." In *An Analytical Approach to the Study of Relics*, edited by Mark Van Strydonck, Jeroen Reyniers, and Fanny Van Cleven, 91–108. Peeters, 2018.

Hashimoto, Akira. "The Invention of a 'Japanese Gheel': Psychiatric Family Care from a Historical and Transnational Perspective." In *Transnational Psychiatries Social and Cultural Histories of Psychiatry in Comparative Perspective, c. 1800–2000*, edited by Ernst Waltraud and Thomas Mueller, 142–71. Cambridge Scholars, 2010.

Hereford Cathedral. "Chained Library." 2023. https://www.herefordcathedral.org/chained-library.

Hoeniger, Cathleen. "The English Gift After the Destruction of the University of Louvain Library in World War I." *Bulletin of the John Rylands Library* 100, no. 1 (2024): 85–112.

Holmes, Catherine, and Naomi Standen. "Introduction: Towards a Global Middle Ages." *Past & Present* 238, no. 13 (2018): 1–44.

Holst, Malin. "Osteological Analysis Coppergate York." York Archaeological Trust For Excavation & Research. York Osteoarchaeology, 2010. https://research.yorkarchaeology.co.uk/wp-content/uploads/2023/08/CoppergateOsteological-Analysis.pdf.

Horden, Peregrine, ed. *Music as Medicine: The History of Music Therapy since Antiquity*. Routledge, 2000.

Houston, Alexandra. "'Seiknes Incurabill': The Evolution of Literary Representations of Leprosy in Medieval and Early Modern English Narratives." *Chicago Journal of History* 7 (2016): 30–41.

Iglesias, Rubén Permuy. "Destruction of Cultural Heritage Is Part of the Strategies of War." *Universitat Oberta de Catalunya*, June 22, 2022. https://www.uoc.edu/en/news/2022/018-gloria-munilla.

Ikram, Muhammad Qaiser, Fazle Hakim Sajjad, and Arash Salardini. "The Head That Wears the Crown: Henry VIII and Traumatic Brain Injury." *Journal of Clinical Neuroscience* 28 (2016): 16–19.

Jones, D. Gareth, and Robyn J. Harris, "Archaeological Human Remains: Scientific, Cultural, and Ethical Considerations." *Current Anthropology* 39, no. 2 (1998): 253–64.

JORVIK Viking Centre. "The People of JORVIK." https://www.jorvikvikingcentre.co.uk/the-vikings/the-people-of-jorvik/.

Kahlow, S. "Prothesen im Mittelalter—ein Überblick aus archäologischer Sicht." In *Homo debilis: Behinderte—Kranke—Versehrte in der Gesellschaft des Mittelalters*, edited by C. Nolte, 201–23. Didymos, 2009.

Kennedy, Amelia. "Crip Time in the Medieval Monasteries." *The Journal of Medieval Monastic Studies* 10 (2021): 67–87.

Kenny, Stephen C. "The Development of Medical Museums in the Antebellum American South: Slave Bodies in Networks of Anatomical Exchange." *Bulletin of the History of Medicine* 87, no. 1 (2013): 32–62.

Kestemont, Mike, et al. "Forgotten Books: The Application of Unseen Species Models to the Survival of Culture." *Science* 375, no. 6582 (2022): 765–69.

Kharoubi, Fatiha, and Hamidi Badra. "Importance of Coins in Historical and Archaeological Studies." *AFAK for Sciences Journal* 10, no. 2 (2025): 254–61.

King, Turi. "We Proved, with 99.999% Certainty, That the Skeleton in the Car Park was Richard III: Here's How." *BBC History Magazine* (2025): 22.

Klein, Cecelia F. "A New Interpretation of the Aztec Statue Called Coatlicue, 'Snakes-Her-Skirt.'" *Ethnohistory* 55, no. 2 (2008): 229–50.

Koenig, Ronnie. "Pregnant Woman Hopes to Stand for All Mothers of Black Men with Powerful Sign." *Today*, June 7, 2020. https://www.today.com/parents/pregnant-woman-hopes-stand-all-mothers-black-men-powerful-sign-t183565, accessed July 6, 2026.

Kowalski, Wojciech. "Legal Status of Human Remains under Polish Cultural Heritage Law." *Santander Art and Culture Law Review* 11, no. 2 (2025): 147–68.

Krause, Heike, Udo Ganslosser, and Nina Marie Hohlfeld. "Dog Training, Keeping and Selection around 1300, Using the Example of Albertus Magnus and Petrus de Crescentiis." *Animals* 13, no. 23 (2023). https://www.mdpi.com/2076-2615/13/23/3698.

KU Leuven. "History of the University Library." May 28, 2024. https://www.kuleuven.be/heritage/collections/history-of-the-university-library.

Ladau, Emily. *Demystifying Disability: What to Know, What to Say, and How to Be an Ally*. Ten Speed, 2021.

Levitas, Andrew S., and Cheryl S. Reid. "An Angel with Down Syndrome in a Sixteenth Century Flemish Nativity Painting." *American Journal of Medical Genetics* 116A, no. 4 (2003): 399–405.

Li, Xiao, et al. "Archaeological and Palaeopathological Study on the Third/Second Century BC Grave from Turfan, China: Individual Health History and Regional Implications," *Quaternary International* 290–91 (2013): 335–43.

Licata, Marta, et al. "Study, Conservation and Exhibition of Human Remains: The Need of a Bioethical Perspective." *Acta Biomed* 91, no. 4 (2020). https://www.mattioli1885journals.com/index.php/actabiomedica/article/view/9674/9371.

Lindquist, Wendi A. "Stealing from the Dead: Scientists, Settlers, and Indian Burial Sites in Early-Nineteenth-Century Oregon." *Oregon Historical Quarterly* 115, no. 3 (2014): 324–43.

Lord, Janet E., and Christopher J. Hart. "Disabled Dead Bodies: Marking the Intersections of International Humanitarian Law and International Human Rights Law." *International Review of the Red Cross* no. 929 (2025): 1–31.

Lou, Michell. "Four Years Ago, An Art Historian Used Lasers to Digitally Map Notre Dame Cathedral. His Work Could Help Save It." *CNN*, April 17, 2019. https://www.cnn.com/style/article/notre-dame-andrew-tallon-laser-scan-trnd/index.html.

Lund, Julie, and Sarah Semple. "Introduction: Medieval Materialities." In *A Cultural History of Objects in the Medieval Ages*, edited by Lund and Semple, 1–28. Bloomsbury, 2021.

MacIsaac, Kristina. "This Pregnant Mother's Protest Sign Is So Powerful." *Motherly*, June 8, 2020. https://www.mother.ly/news/this-pregnant-moms-protest-sign-is-so-powerful, accessed 6 July 2026.

Manatakis, Lexi. "Harmonia Rosales Repaints Classic Artworks to Show God is a Black Woman." *Dazed*, September 5, 2018. https://www.dazeddigital.com/art-photography/article/41202/1/harmonia-rosales-repaints-classic-artworks-god-is-a-black-woman-rjd-gallery.

Martinez-Frias, Maria Luisa. "The Real Earliest Historical Evidence of Down Syndrome." *American Journal of Medical Genetics* 132A, no. 2 (2005): 231.

Maxwell Museum of Anthropology. "Iconoclasm: Questions of Veneration, Destruction and Power." *The University of New Mexico*, 2020. https://maxwellmuseum.unm.edu/sites/default/files/public/online-exhibits/Iconoclasm%20July%2016%20 2020%20The%20Maxwell%20Museum%20of%20Anthropology.pdf.

McCrary, Lorraine Krall. "Geel's Family Care Tradition: Care, Communities, and the Social Inclusion of Persons with Disabilities." *Journal of Literary and Cultural Disability Studies* 11, no. 3 (2017): 285–301.

Mfoafo-M'Carthy, Magnus, Jeff Grischow, and Festus Moasun. *Experiencing Disability Stigma in Ghana*. Lexington, 2024.

Micarelli, Ileana, et al. "Survival to Amputation in Pre-Antibiotic Era: A Case Study from a Longobard Necropolis (6th–8th Centuries AD)." *Journal of Anthropological Sciences* 96 (2018): 1–16.

Milne, Krista A. "Guide Dogs in Medieval Art and Writing." *Dr. Krista A. Milne*. https://kristamurchison.com/medieval-guide-dogs/.

Mohatt, Nathaniel. "Historical Trauma as Public Narrative: A Conceptual Review of How History Impacts Present-day Health." *Soc Sci Med* 106 (2014): 128–36.

Mortensen, Lars Boje. "Why Ancient and Medieval Texts Are Intangible Cultural Heritage." *University of Southern Denmark*, 2020. https://www.sdu.dk/en/forskning/cml/news/blog_lars_2020, accessed July 6, 2026.

Murphy, Fiona. "Aboriginal Sign Languages Have Been Used for Thousands of Years." *ABC News*, June 18, 2021. https://www.abc.net.au/news/2021-06-19/australian-indigenous-sign-languages/100185504.

Nakamura, Osamu. "Family Care of Mentally Ill Patients." *Indian Journal of Social Psychiatry* 22, no. 3–4, (2006): 98–103.

National Down Syndrome Society. "About Down Syndrome." 2025. https://ndss.org/about, accessed January 3, 2026.

National Institute of Arthritis and Musculoskeletal and Skin Diseases. "Paget's Disease of Bone," September 2022. https://www.niams.nih.gov/health-topics/pagets-disease-bone.

National Institute of Neurological Disorders and Stroke. "Traumatic Brain Injury (TBI)." https://www.ninds.nih.gov/health-information/disorders/traumatic-brain-injury-tbi.

National Organization for Rare Disorders. "Arthrogryposis Multiplex Congenita." November 11, 2024. https://rarediseases.org/rare-diseases/arthrogryposis-multiplex-congenita/.

National Scoliosis Foundation. "Information and Support." https://www.scoliosis.org/info.php, accessed July 6, 2026.

Negussie, Tesfaye. "Mother of Sinzae Reed, Black 13-Year-Old Killed in Ohio, Demands Justice." *ABCNews*, January 6, 2023. https://abcnews.go.com/US/mother-sinzae-reed-black-13-year-killed-ohio/story?id=96134953.

Nesbitt, John W. and Timothy S. Miller. *Walking Corpses: Leprosy in Byzantium and the Medieval West*. Cornell University Press, 2023.

NewsOne Staff. "147 Black Men and Boys Killed by Police." *NEWSONE*, June 12, 2023. https://newsone.com/playlist/black-men-boys-who-were-killed-by-police/item/68.

Nolan, Blair, et al. "Disability and Care in Late Medieval Lund, Sweden: An Analysis of Trauma and Intersecting Identities, Aided by Photogrammetric Digitization and Visualization." *Open Archaeology* 11, no. 1 (2025): 1–18.

Novak, Shannon A. "Battle-Related Trauma." In *Blood Red Roses: The Archaeology of a Mass Grave from the Battle of Towton AD 1461*, edited by Veronica Fiorato, Anthea Boylston, and Christopher Knüsel, 90–102. Oxbow, 2007.

Nuut, Sander, et, al., "Pets or Functional Animals: Dogs and Cats in Medieval and Early Modern Estonia." *Estonian Journal of Archaeology* 27, 3S (2023): 83–104.

Ostermeier, Mark. "History of Guide Dog Use by Veterans." *Military Medicine* 175, no. 8 (2010): 587–93.

OxfordUnion. "Black Lives Matter: Stories from the Mothers | Oxford Union." *YouTube*, January 4, 2017. https://youtu.be/lZuzRMMdgYo.

Our Lady of Czestochowa Foundation. *The Glories of Czestochowa and Jasna Gora: Miracles Attributed to Our Lady's Intercession*. Marian, 2004.

Pasierb, Janusz. *The Shrine of the Black Madonna at Czestochowa*. Interpress, 1989.

Phillips, Gervase. "The Employment of War Dogs in the Medieval and Early Modern West." *British Journal for Military History* 7, no. 1 (2021): 2–20.

Potok, Bryan. "Prosthetic Legs Don't Give Athletes Unfair Advantage—Study." *Amputee Store*, March 15, 2022. https://amputeestore.com/blogs/amputee-life/prosthetic-running-legs-dont-give-adaptive-athletes-unfair-advantage.

Půtová, Barbora. "Freak Shows: Otherness of the Human Body as a Form of Public Presentation." *Anthropologie* 56, no. 2 (2018): 91–102.

Ralston, S. H. "Paget's Disease of Bone." *The New England Journal of Medicine* 368, no. 7 (2013): 644–50.

Rayner, Emma. "AncientBiotics—A Medieval Remedy for Modern Day Superbugs?" *The University of Nottingham*, March 30, 2015. https://www.nottingham.ac.uk/news/pressreleases/2015/march/ancientbiotics---a-medieval-remedy-for-modern-day-superbugs.aspx.

Reilly, Maura. *Curatorial Activism: Towards an Ethics of Curating*. Thames & Hudson, 2018.

Rice, Nicole R. *The Medieval Hospital: Literary Culture and Community in England, 1350–1550*. Notre Dame University Press, 2023.

Rivollat, Maïté, et al. "Ancient Down Syndrome: An Osteological Case from Saint-Jean-des-Vignes, Northeastern France, from the 5–6th Century." *International Journal of Paleopathology* 7 (2014): 8–14.

Robb, John, et al. "Osteobiography: The History of the Body as Real Bottom-Line History." *Bioarchaeology International* 3, no. 1 (2019): 16–31.

Rohde, Eleanour Sinclair. *The Old English Herbals*. Longmans, Green, 1922.

Rossillo, Amanda. "Contemplating the Lives behind Ancient Bones." *Scientific American*, June 19, 2019. https://www.scientificamerican.com/blog/observations/contemplating-the-lives-behind-ancient-bones/, accessed December 30, 2025.

Row-Heyveld, Lindsey. *Dissembling Disability in Early Modern English Drama*. Palgrave Macmillan, 2018.

"Safeguarding Foster Care Heritage in the Merciful City of Geel: A Community-based Care Model." *UNESCO Intangible Cultural Heritage*. https://ich.unesco.org/en/BSP/safeguarding-foster-care-heritage-in-the-merciful-city-of-geel-a-community-based-care-model-00622.

Sajjadi, S. M. S., M. Casanova, L. Costantini, and K. O. Lorentz. "Sistan and Baluchistan Project: Short Reports on the Tenth Campaign of Excavations at Shahr-I Sokhta," *Iran: Journal of the British Institute of Persian Studies* 46, no. 1 (2008): 307–34.

Sandell, Richard, et al. "In the Shadow of the Freakshow: The Impact of Freakshow Tradition on the Display and Understanding of Disability History in Museums." *Disability Studies Quarterly* 25, no. 4 (2005): https://dsq-sds.org/article/id/5613/.

Schlich, Thomas. "The 'Bionic Men' of World War I." *CNN*, June 27, 2014. https://www.cnn.com/2014/06/26/opinion/schlich-world-war-i-prosthetics/index.html.

Scovazzi, Tullio. "Human Remains as Cultural Heritage." In *The Routledge Handbook of Heritage and the Law*, edited by Lucas Lixinski and Lucie K. Morisset, 456–72. Routledge, 2024.

Skinner, Patricia. *Living with Disfigurement in Early Medieval Europe*. Palgrave, 2017.

Solomon, Andrew. *The Noonday Demon: An Atlas of Depression*. Scriber, 2015.

Spencer-Hall, Alicia. "Stopping the Clock(s): Precarious Times in the Academy." *Medieval, She Wrote*, September 16, 2019. https://www.medievalshewrote.com/blog/2019/9/15/stopping-the-clocks-precarious-times-in-the-academy, accessed 6 July 2026.

Starbuck, John M. "On the Antiquity of Trisomy 21: Moving Towards a Quantitative Diagnosis of Down Syndrome in Historic Material Culture." *Journal of Contemporary Anthropology* 2, no. 1 (2011): 19–44.

Stewart, Jessica. "Mini Sculptures in Front of Monuments Help Visually Impaired People Explore Architecture." *My Modern MET*, November 11, 2019. https://mymodernmet.com/bronze-scale-models-visually-impaired/.

Sutherland, Tim. "Introduction." *Towton Battlefield Archaeology Project*. http://towtonbattle.free.fr/, accessed January 1, 2026.

Sveinsdóttir, Hólmfríður. "A Material Culture of Medieval Disability: Contextualising Norwegian Votive Offerings." *Norwegian Archaeological Review* 57, no. 1 (2024): 39–58.

Teboh, Consoler. "Mental Health Inequities in Africa: A Human Rights Perspective." *Expanding Perspectives on Human Rights in Africa* (2019): 193–215.

Tracy, Kisha. *Why Study the Middle Ages?* Arc Humanities, 2022.

"Trauma and Violence." Substance Abuse and Mental Health Services Administration, https://www.samhsa.gov/trauma-violence. Qtd. in "Achieving Behavioral Health Equity for Children, Families, and Communities: Proceedings of a Workshop." *National Library of Medicine*, 2019. https://www.ncbi.nlm.nih.gov/books/NBK540764.

Unites Access. "History of the Term 'Handicapped.'" May 28, 2024. https://www.unitedaccess.com/us/en/blog/disability-rights/history-of-term-handicapped.html.

United Nations Educational, Scientific, and Cultural Organization. "Cultural Heritage." UNESCO Glossary, 2009. https://databrowser.uis.unesco.org/resources/glossary/2488.

van Bilsen, Hench P. J. G. "Lessons to Be Learned from the Oldest Community Psychiatric Service in the World: Geel in Belgium." *BJPsych Bulletin* 40 (2016): 207–11.

van Daal, Jan. "Prevention, Breakage, Care: Anticipating Damage in Medieval Art Technology." Work in Progress. The Artists' Gestures and Skills Explored through Art Technological Source Research. Proceedings of the Ninth Symposium of the ICOM-CC Working Group on Art Technological Source Research, November 24–25, 2022. 2025. Academia.edu. https://www.academia.edu/143622596/Prevention_breakage_care_anticipating_damage_in_Medieval_art_technology.

Wagoner, Brady, and Ignacio Brescó de Luna. "Collective Grief: Mourning Rituals, Politics and Memorial Sites." In *Cultural, Existential and Phenomenological Dimensions of Grief Experience*, edited by Allan Køster and Ester Holte Kofod, 197–213. Routledge, 2021.

Walker-Meikle, Kathleen. *Medieval Pets*. Boydell & Brewer, 2012.

Waugaman, Richard M. "Traumatic Brain Injury as One Possible Cause of King Henry VIII's Morbid Obesity and Truculence." *Notes and Queries* 66 [264], no. 3 (2019): 374–75.

Weinstein, Philip. "Palaeopathology by Proxy: The Case of Egil's Bones." *Journal of Archaeological Science* 34, no. 7 (2005): 1077–82.

Wheatley, Edward. *Stumbling Blocks Before the Blind: Medieval Constructions of a Disability: Medieval Constructions of Disability*. University of Michigan Press, 2010.

Windmuller-Luna, Kristen. "Ethiopian Healing Scrolls." *Heilbrunn Timeline of Art History*, The Metropolitan Museum of Art, 2015. https://www.metmuseum.org/essays/ethiopian-healing-scrolls.

Wollina, Uwe, et al. "Leprosy in the Middle Ages: A European Perspective." *Clinics in Dermatology* 43, no. 3 (2025): 431–39.

World Health Organization. "Disability." March 7, 2023. https://www.who.int/newsroom/fact-sheets/detail/disability-and-health.

Yağcı, Gözde, and Nilgün Bek. "A Historical Perspective of the Management of Scoliosis." *Erciyes Medical Journal* 44, no. 4 (2022): 439–46.

(All URLs were accessed on July 6, 2026.)

INDEX

DOI: 10.17302/asgs326810 © Arc Humanities Press